#2141

S0-AAG-356

# Therapeutic
# Medications
## IN
# Sports Medicine

# Therapeutic Medications
## IN
## Sports Medicine

**Malissa Martin, EdD, ATC**

Assistant Professor
Director, Athletic Training Program
Department of Physical Education
University of South Carolina
Columbia, South Carolina

**William N. Yates, Jr, PhD, RPh**

YAK Inc.
Columbia, South Carolina

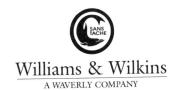

Williams & Wilkins
A WAVERLY COMPANY

BALTIMORE • PHILADELPHIA • LONDON • PARIS • BANGKOK
BUENOS AIRES • HONG KONG • MUNICH • SYDNEY • TOKYO • WROCLAW

*Editor:* Eric P. Johnson
*Managing Editor:* Linda S. Napora
*Marketing Manager:* Christine Kushner
*Production Coordinator:* Marette Magargle-Smith
*Project Editor:* Jennifer D. Weir
*Designer:* Graphic World Publishing Services
*Typesetter:* Peirce Graphic Services, Inc.
*Printer/Binder:* Vicks Lithograph & Printing Corp.

Copyright © 1998 Williams & Wilkins

351 West Camden Street
Baltimore, Maryland 21201-2436 USA

Rose Tree Corporate Center
1400 North Providence Road
Building II, Suite 5025
Media, Pennsylvania 19063-2043 USA

**Disclaimer:** The information in this reference guide is to supplement the knowledge of athletic trainers and other athletic health care providers concerning therapeutic medications and sports medicine. This information is advisory only and is not intended to replace sound clinical judgment or individual care in the delivery of athletic health care services. The user of this information assumes sole responsibility for decisions and actions taken based upon the information in this guide.

All rights reserved. This book is protected by copyright. No part of this book may be reproduced in any form or by any means, including photocopying, or utilized by any information storage and retrieval system without written permission from the copyright owner.

Accurate indications, adverse reactions, and dosage schedules for drugs are provided in this book, but it is possible that they may change. The reader is urged to review the package information data of the manufacturers of the medications mentioned.

*Printed in the United States of America*

**Library of Congress Cataloging-in-Publication Data**

Martin, Malissa.
  Therapeutic medications in sports medicine / Malissa Martin, William N. Yates, Jr.
      p.    cm.
  Includes index.
  ISBN 0-683-30223-X
  1. Drugs.   2. Sports medicine.   3. Sports injuries.   4. Chemotherapy.   I. Yates, William N.   II. Title.
  [DNLM: 1. Athletic Injuries—drug therapy.   QT 261 M382t 1998]
  RM301.M376   1998
  6159.19088796—dc21
  DNLM/DLC
  for Library of Congress                                            97-45783
                                                                          CIP

*The publishers have made every effort to trace the copyright holders for borrowed material. If they have inadvertently overlooked any, they will be pleased to make the necessary arrangements at the first opportunity.*

To purchase additional copies of this book, call our customer service department at **(800) 638-0672** or fax orders to **(800) 447-8438**. For other book services, including chapter reprints and large quantity sales, ask for the Special Sales department.

Canadian customers should call **(800) 665-1148**, or fax **(800) 665-0103**. For all other calls originating outside of the United States, please call **(410) 528-4223** or fax us at **(410) 528-8550**.

**Visit Williams & Wilkins on the Internet: http://www.wwilkins.com** or contact our customer service department at **custserv@wwilkins.com**. Williams & Wilkins customer service representatives are available from 8:30 am to 6:00 pm, EST, Monday through Friday, for telephone access.

                                                                98 99 00 01 02
                                                                1 2 3 4 5 6 7 8 9 10

This guide has been prepared to serve as a quick reference to therapeutic medications used in the treatment of common injuries and illnesses of the physically active population. It is directed to athletic trainers, physical therapists, school nurses, physician assistants, physical therapist aides, and health care professionals who work with all ages and levels of the physically active population (youth, recreational, high school, college, and professional athletes). The guide acquaints the user with the therapeutic medications most often used for injury and illnesses associated with sports medicine and the physically active population.

There are four sections along with appendices, glossary, references, and index. Section I is the User's Guide and provides brief instructions on how best to use the guide. Section II introduces the reader to general information and precautions for all drugs and should be reviewed prior to using the guide. Common terms and definitions are found in the glossary. Common medical abbreviations are found on the inside cover for quick reference when reading drug information in Section IV. Becoming familiar with the terms, definitions, and common medical abbreviations enhances use of the guide. Section III reviews legal considerations for the administration and dispensing of therapeutic medications. Record-keeping procedures are discussed as well. Appendix B provides some sample forms for record-keeping procedures in the documentation of over-the-counter medications.

Section IV presents common therapeutic drugs used in the treatment of injuries and illnesses of the physically active population. This section is arranged by drug classification. Each classification includes common medications listed by their generic and brand names, the medication's action, indications for use, side effects, warnings, dosing information, and notes containing additional information unique to each medication. Notes may include a medication's relationship to physical activity and will indicate if the medication is a National Collegiate Athletic Association (NCAA) and or United State Olympic Committee (USOC) banned substance.

# ACKNOWLEDGMENTS

The idea for this guide was initiated through the work of Beth Sloan and Jan Salis. They developed a *Physicians' Desk Reference for Athletic Training* while completing their master's work at Indiana State University in the 1980s. Since then, I (M.M.) have used their reference throughout my clinical and academic work. I want to personally thank Beth and Jan for providing me with the groundwork to pursue and develop this reference book.

The authors also acknowledge the students who were in the *Alcohol, Other Drugs, and the Athlete* course at the University of South Carolina in the Department of Physical Education during the summers of 1994 and 1995. It was through their initial efforts that the foundation of this guide was developed and completed. A special thanks to Joseph Crawford, Rita Wilburn-Gassert, Carol Jawoski, Tom Kaufmann, Chris Sea, and Julyanne Shiflett.

A project such as this is not possible without critical reviews and guidance from colleagues in the field. A special thanks is extended to Marje Albohm, Herb Amato, Pat Aronson, Patsy Huff, and Jamie Moul for their timely efforts.

In addition, sincere appreciation is extended to Donna Balado and Jennifer Schmidt who initially worked with the development of the book. We also acknowledge Eric Johnson for his humor, which was encouraging through the progressive frustrations, along with Linda Napora and others at Williams & Wilkins who provided direction and saw the book through publication. Your talents and support have been consistently and appreciatively unconditional. Thank you.

Malissa Martin
Bill Yates

# CONTENTS

## APPENDICES

## GLOSSARY

# User's Guide

*Therapeutic Medications in Sports Medicine* is a guide to assist athletic trainers and other health care professionals who work with athletes and physically active persons in situations where the participant is using a medication and it is necessary to understand the indication(s) that resulted in use of the medication and how this medication may affect the individual's performance.

To keep this guide concise and quick to use, not all medications are included. Drugs utilized primarily in institutional settings (i.e., hospitals and nursing homes) and medications used in rare diseases are not included. There are over 70,000 nonprescription products available and over 400 different nonprescription ingredients; this guide focuses on the most common ingredients and brand names of drugs used for the treatment of athletic-related injuries and illnesses. It is important to carefully read the ingredients contained in a product. Brand names cannot be utilized to indicate what a product may contain. Many brand names now have several formulas, each containing various medications in different combinations.

To best use this guide, review Sections II and III and the Glossary. Become familiar with terms and definitions. In addition to the presentation of legal concerns and issues when using therapeutic medications, Section III suggests record-keeping procedures. Samples of record-keeping forms, which should be used at all times for documentation and accountability purposes, are found in Appendix B.

Section IV provides the bulk of the text. For the most efficient use of this guide, refer to the index to locate the drug (generic and brand names are included) in question. The index will provide the page number. Drugs can also be found within each pharmacological classification. For example, if the drug naproxen sodium is in question and you know it is a nonsteroidal anti-inflammatory, refer to the table of contents under Analgesics, NSAIDs (nonsteroidal anti-inflammatory drugs); turn to that category and you will find naproxen sodium in the alphabetized list of NSAIDs. Of course, you will also find it in the index.

Once you have located the drug, you will find essential information organized (in most cases) as follows:

- Action—what the drug does
- Indication—why the drug should be used
- Banned Substances—whether the drug contains ingredients banned by the NCAA and/or USOC
- Name of drug (bold type = generic; italic type = brand name; ℞ = prescription drug)
- Side Effects
- Warnings
- Dosing
- Notes

Refer to the sample page for a step-by-step explanation of the format.

Description of Table Format

## ❶Nonsteroidal Anti-Inflammatory Drugs (NSAIDs)

❷ **ACTION** NSAIDs work by reducing inflammation (pain, swelling, redness, heat) and by inhibiting chemicals in the body that produce tissue irritation and cause inflammation.

❸ **INDICATION** Used for pain, fever, anti-inflammatory effects, and arthritis pain relief. NSAIDs are also used for mild to moderate pain resulting from conditions such as headache, dental pain, athletic injury, menstrual cramps, flu, colds, and sore throats. They may also be prescribed for rheumatoid arthritis, sunburn, gouty arthritis, ankylosing spondylitis, bursitis, tendinitis, osteoarthritis, and migraine headaches..

| ❹ Generic Name / *Brand Name* | Side Effects ❺ | Warnings ❻ | Dosing ❼ | Notes ❽ |
|---|---|---|---|---|
| **Diclofenac Potassium** | Stomach upset, ulceration, drowsiness, dizziness, blurred vision, sensitivity to sunlight. | Avoid aspirin and alcoholic beverages, which can increase the risk for stomach upset and ulceration. | Take with food. | |
| **Ibuprofen** *Advil, Motrin IB* more tablets or caplets (OTC) *Children's Motrin* Suspension (OTC) *Motrin, Rufen* tablets (℞) | Stomach upset, ulceration, drowsiness, dizziness, blurred vision, sensitivity to sunlight. | Avoid aspirin and alcoholic beverages, which can increase the risk for stomach upset and ulceration. | Take with food. | OTC Use—Do not take for than 3 days for fever or 10 days for pain. |

| Generic Name<br>*Brand Name* | Side Effects | Warnings | Dosing | Notes |
|---|---|---|---|---|
| **Naproxen Sodium**<br>*Aleve* tablets<br>or caplet (OTC)<br>*Anaprox, Anaprox DS*<br>tablets (℞) | Stomach upset, ulceration, drowsiness, dizziness, blurred vision, sensitivity to sunlight. | Avoid aspirin and alcoholic beverages, which can increase the risk for stomach upset and ulceration. | Take with food. | OTC Use—Do not take more than 3 days for fever or 10 days for pain, and do not take more than 3 tablets in 24 hours. |

❶ General drug category/classification.

❷ Action—Brief description of how the medication works in the body for this drug category.

❸ Indication—Symptoms for which these medications are prescribed. This does not include all unapproved indications. Unique indications for a medication may be found under "Notes."

❹ Generic name for medication is in bold type. When a medication has multiple ingredients, the generic name will consist of two or more names separated by commas. Brand name for medication is listed in italic type. When two or more brands are listed, they are separated by commas. Prescription status of the medication is denoted with the following abbreviations:

OTC—available without a prescription (over-the-counter)
℞—requires a prescription
C-II—Schedule II controlled substance
C-III—Schedule III controlled substance
C-IV—Schedule IV controlled substance
C-V—Schedule V controlled substance

❺ Side effects—General side effects of the medication. This is not a comprehensive list, but a guideline for the most common side effects and those most likely to affect athletic performance.

❻ Warnings—Crucial aspects of reactions to medications. These focus on common problems that may occur.

❼ Dosing—Activities of consuming the medication; this information can affect the treatment because it may determine the effectiveness of the medication.

❽ Notes—Additional information unique to that particular medication.

Common medical abbreviations are defined on the inside cover for easy reference. The Glossary contains common terms and definitions that are helpful in understanding and using the information provided in Section IV.

Finally, the appendices provide handy reference information:

Appendix A:  Schedule of Controlled Substances

Appendix B:  Record-keeping forms

Appendix C:  Poison control information and centers

# General Information and Precautions

## GENERAL INFORMATION

### Proper Use

- Medications should be taken only as directed
- If medication is not effective, consult a physician or pharmacist
- Medications should not be taken together before consulting a physician or pharmacist
- Labels should not be removed from medication bottles or containers
- Medications should not be used past the expiration date marked on the container. Some medications become toxic while others loose potency.
- Tablets, capsules, or liquids that look discolored should not be taken
- Medications should never be taken if tampering is evident
- Oral medications should be taken with a full glass of water unless directed otherwise
- Medication should be taken with food if directions indicate
- Specially marked measuring spoons or caps should be used when measuring liquid medications
- Skin patches should be applied directly to clean, dry skin with little or no hair
- Skin patches should be rotated to different areas of the skin to prevent skin irritation
- All directions should be closely followed when using respiratory inhalers
- Medications should never be shared with another person
- Prior to receiving medication or prior to surgery, all other current medications should be reported to the physician

- If an overdose has been taken, the nearest poison control center should be called immediately

### Medications and Traveling

- Medications should be carried by the athletic trainer or patient rather than in a stored bag or checked luggage
- Take a large enough supply to cover emergency situations while on the road
- Plan ahead and make sure there is a source of medication while traveling
- Take a copy of a written prescription
- Keep medications in the original container for identification purposes
- Keep medications in a safe and secure place

### Storing Medications

- Always keep medications out of the reach of children and pets
- Keep medications in a locked cabinet or safe and secure place
- Keep medications in the original container
- Store medications away from heat, direct light, and damp places, and keep from freezing
- Do not keep outdated medications
- Non-child-resistant caps can be requested on prescription medications

### Information on a Prescription Container*

Patient's name
Pharmacy name, address, and telephone number
Name of medication
Dose information and direction for use
Number of refills (if any)
Warnings (if any)
Date prescription was filled
Name of person who dispensed the medication
*Individual state laws may require that additional information be on the container

### Seven-Point Label for Over-the-Counter Medications

Name of product
Name and address of manufacturer

Net contents
Name and quantity of active ingredients
Name of habit-forming drugs
Cautions and warnings
Adequate directions for safe and effective use

## GENERAL PRECAUTIONS

### Alcohol

Alcohol is a depressant and can increase or decrease effects of other drugs such as intensifying the effects of sedative drugs (i.e., drowsiness). The amount of alcohol may not be as important as its chemical reaction. Because alcohol is used in many liquid preparations to dissolve medication, it is important to consider the presence of alcohol in both prescription and nonprescription products. Often, warnings concerning the use of alcohol while taking a certain drug are listed on the drug product.

### Drugs and Food

Food can interfere or assist with the absorption of a drug and can limit nausea and other stomach side effects. Drugs can increase or decrease the appetite. Some drugs may also decrease the absorption of certain body nutrients such as vitamins or minerals. It is important to follow all directions when taking a drug, especially if the prescription requires the drug to be taken with food or before or after meals.

### Drugs and the Environment

Drugs can affect physiological functions such as sweating, salivation, urination, and bowel movements, which in turn can affect the ability of the body to regulate and control body temperature. Medications can cause retention or loss of fluids resulting in dehydration or edema. This can affect the ability of participation at different levels of exercise and can place a person at risk of more severe problems such as heat illness.

### Drugs and the Sunlight

Many drugs possess the potential to make an individual more susceptible to the ultraviolet rays of the sun. This results in a shorter time span needed for symptoms such as burning, rash, or allergies to the sun to occur. It is recommended that exposure to sunlight and sunlamps be limited, and that a proper level of sunscreen be used if medications indicate sun sensitivity.

## Drugs and Allergies

Allergies to medications are common, unpredictable, and sometimes life threatening. Previous safe use of a medication does not guarantee that an allergic reaction will not occur with subsequent use. Allergies to one drug increase the potential of allergy to other chemically related drugs. Allergic reaction symptoms include rash, itching, difficult breathing, and anaphylactic reaction. Even mild allergic reactions may require immediate medical attention.

## Drugs and Side Effects

Side effects of medications may be related to the dose and duration of the drug therapy as well as current use of other medications. Many side effects are temporary and dissipate within a few hours or days of starting the medication. Other side effects may not occur for days or weeks into the therapy. Not all side effects are listed in this publication. The focus in this publication is on side effects that are most likely to occur or those that may affect athletic performance and physical activity. Caution should be exercised in concluding that a side effect is caused by a particular medication. Often side effects may be the result of other factors (e.g., drowsiness may result from exercise-induced fatigue).

The existence of a side effect must be balanced with the benefit of the drug versus the possibility of changing the drug treatment. Some side effects can be managed by changing the time or administration of medication, or treating the side effect with another medication.

## Mixing Medications

The prescribing physician or pharmacist should be consulted with questions concerning interactive effects of both prescription and nonprescription medications. Medications can counteract each other or become additive in effect. For example, medications that may cause drowsiness when used together (with synergistic) may increase the effect of drowsiness as compared with when the medications are used alone. Decongestants can increase blood pressure reducing the effectiveness of medications used to decrease blood pressure.

## Completing the Dosage

It is important to follow directions to complete a dosage regimen. It is important to complete the prescribed dose of medication especially with drugs such as antibiotics and antifungals. Incomplete therapy can result in developing a resistance to the medication and a recurrence of the infection. Other medications, such as corticosteroids and seizure medications, may need to be tapered to prevent adverse effects.

## Children and Elderly

Physiologically, children and the elderly may react differently to drugs than adults in general. Children may have the opposite reaction of adults (e.g., a medication that may cause drowsiness in adults may cause hyperactivity or irritability in children). Elderly patients may have reduced body fat and muscle levels that affect the absorption and distribution of drugs in the body. This may increase the side effects and or toxicity of a drug.

Some drugs have been studied as to the effect in children and the elderly. Nonprescription medications generally have dosage information for adults and children over a certain age.

## Pregnancy

Many medications should not be used during pregnancy, especially in the first 3 months. Women should consult their primary care physician prior to using any prescription or over-the-counter medication during pregnancy. Warnings for use of drugs during pregnancy are not included in this guide.

## Breast Feeding

Drugs may be excreted into breast milk and consequently be absorbed by the infant. Dependency on any drug could affect the nursing child. Women who are breast feeding should consult their physician or pharmacist. Warnings for the use of drugs while breast feeding are not included in this guide.

## Drug Overdose

A drug overdose occurs when a lethal or toxic amount of a drug is taken. It is usually the result of taking too large a dose or too many doses. Signs and symptoms of drug overdose can be dependent on the type of drug and the adverse effects of that drug. These effects can be exhibited as excessive drowsiness, cyanosis, difficulty in breathing, chest pains, stupor, confusion, and visual disturbances. If overdose is suspected, immediate medical attention is required. Do not use items such as Ipecac or other vomit-inducing agents unless directed by a physician. Refer to Appendix C for a listing of poison control centers.

## Potential Misuse by Athletes

Athletes may misuse prescription medications due to a lack of knowledge and misinformation. It is imperative that athletes receive both oral and verbal information when given drugs. A category of drugs often misused by athletes is NSAIDs. Athletes use NSAIDs for both their anti-inflammatory and analgesic effects. Too often, however, athletes take NSAIDs too frequently and in greater quantities than recommended. The practice of "more is better" is often the case. Overtaking NSAIDs can have adverse effects on the gastrointestinal tract, liver, and kidneys.

Another potential misuse of medications by athletes is combining medications with alcohol. Alcohol can decrease the effects of some medications and can also cause toxicity. Medications should never be mixed with other chemicals or drugs unless the combination has been authorized by a pharmacist or physician.

## Banned Drugs

The National Collegiate Athletic Association (NCAA) and the United States Olympic Committee (USOC) have established a list of medications that are banned from use in athletes. Use of these drugs can result in disqualification from event participation. The banned drugs are not the same for both organizations. Always consult a current list when this is an issue. For information concerning banned drugs list:
NCAA, PO Box 1906, Mission, KS 66201
USOC Drug Hotline      1-800-233-0393

*It is recommended that persons check with state boards of pharmacy and medical boards for the most up-to-date individual state regulations on the administration and dispensing of medications.*

# Legal Considerations and Record-Keeping Procedures

Athletic trainers often provide suggestions to athletes concerning types of medications to use for various injuries and or illnesses. It is illegal for an athletic trainer to dispense medications. The dispensing of medications is defined as providing both prescription and over-the-counter medications to a person beyond a single dose. An example of dispensing medications is an athletic trainer providing a 1-week supply of ibuprofen to an athlete or a 3-day supply of erythromycin. Pharmacists and physicians can dispense medications. In some states, nurse practitioners and physician assistants can dispense medications. *In addition, physicians cannot instruct an athletic trainer to dispense medications.*

Athletic trainers can, however, administer nonprescription medications. The administration of medications is defined as providing one dose of a medication for immediate use. An example of administering a medication is an athletic trainer providing an athlete with a single dose of ibuprofen. They cannot provide prescription medications unless they have been prescribed by a physician and dispensed by a recognized professional (e.g., a pharmacist).

## GUIDELINES FOR NONPRESCRIPTION MEDICATIONS

How can athletic trainers safely keep medications and provide them to athletes? The following are suggested guidelines to use when keeping medications in the athletic training room.

- do not keep prescription medications in the athletic training room
- if prescription medications are required by the team physician, keep them in the physician's bag or in a separate cabinet that is locked at all times and in no way available to athletes, students, or other persons. Controlled substances are the sole responsibility of the team physician

- dispensing of medications must be done only by a properly licensed person
- all medications should be properly stored according to storage recommendations for each medication
- nonprescription medications should be kept in a locked cabinet and not on tables and counters for athletes to take at will
- discard all medications the expiration date of which has passed
- inventory medications on a regular basis
- work in concert with the team physician and area pharmacist when ordering and purchasing nonprescription medications
- all emergency and travel kits containing prescription and nonprescription medications should be routinely inspected for drug quality, security, and expiration dates
- all nonprescription medications given to athletes should be recorded
- medication reference materials should be available
- patient education should be available either through written or verbal means (verbal is required by law in most states)
- follow-up should be performed to ensure athlete is complying with drug regimen and to know if drug therapy is effective for the prescribed condition

## GUIDELINES FOR RECORD-KEEPING

All medications given to athletes should be documented through a recording system. Records should include the following information:
- name of athlete and sport in which the athlete participates
- date
- name of drug and dose given
- signature of person who provided the medication

Records can be kept through a paper or computer system. Examples of record-keeping documentation are in Appendix B. Recording of prescription medication should be done by the team physician.

# Commonly Used Drugs

## Analgesics

### Acetaminophen

**ACTION** Reduces fever by directly acting on the hypothalamic heat-regulating center to increase heat dissipation. The analgesic effect is unclear.

**INDICATION** For the use of fever and pain. Acetaminophen does not reduce swelling and inflammation.

| Generic Name<br>*Brand Name* | Side Effects | Warnings | Dosing | Notes |
|---|---|---|---|---|
| **Acetaminophen (APAP)**<br>*Children's Tylenol, Tempra* chewable tablet, solution (OTC)<br>*Children's Tylenol* suspension, syrup (OTC)<br>*Tylenol* tablet, caplet, gelcap (OTC)<br>*Feverall* suppository (OTC) | Anemia, skin eruptions, jaundice. | Do not use for more than 5 days for pain or swelling or 3 days for fever without consulting with a physician. | Do not exceed daily dose of 4 grams per day including what may be received in other medication products containing acetaminophen. | Chronic use and/or high doses can lead to liver and kidney problems. |

## Antirheumatic Agents

**ACTION** Antirheumatic agents reduce the joint swelling and inflammation.

**INDICATION** Used to treat rheumatoid arthritis. These agents are generally reserved for individuals unresponsive to other more conservative treatments.

| Generic Name<br>*Brand Name* | Side Effects | Warnings | Dosing | Notes |
|---|---|---|---|---|
| **Auranofin**<br>*Ridaura*<br>capsule (℞) | Sore mouth, indigestion, metallic taste, nose bleeds, rash, itching. | Observe good oral hygiene during treatment. Regular follow-up with a physician is important to monitor for side effects. | | May also be prescribed for psoriatic arthritis. |
| **Hydroxychloro-quine**<br>*Plaquenil Sulfate*<br>tablet (℞) | Vision problems, hearing loss, sore throat, unusual bleeding or bruising, itching or rash, muscle weakness, mood changes. | Notify physician of side effects. Regular follow-up with a physician, including blood counts, is important to monitor for side effects. | Take with food or milk to avoid GI upset. | Also used for acute malarial attacks and lupus erythematosus. |
| **Methotrexate**<br>*Rheumatrex*<br>tablet (℞) | Blurred vision, sore throat, mouth sores, unusual bleeding or bruising, black stools, swelling of legs, skin rash. | May cause drowsiness. Avoid alcohol, which may increase side effects. Contact physician if side effects experienced. | Take with food or milk to avoid GI upset. Dose is taken on a weekly, not daily basis. | Regular follow-up with a physician, including blood counts, is important to monitor for side effects. |

## Central Analgesics

**ACTION** Although action is not understood, this medication produce analgesia with significantly less respiratory depression than morphine.

**INDICATION** Used for moderate to moderately severe pain.

| Generic Name<br>*Brand Name* | Side Effects | Warnings | Dosing | Notes |
|---|---|---|---|---|
| **Tramadol**<br>*Ultram* tablet (℞) | Drowsiness, dizziness, confusion, nausea, vomiting, constipation, appetite loss, dry mouth. | Avoid alcohol, other depressants, and drowsiness-causing drugs. | May take with or without food. | May take 1 to 2 hours to work. |

## Gout Agents

**ACTION** Gout agents work either by reducing the formation of uric acid in the body or by decreasing the inflammatory response to uric acid.

**INDICATION** Used to treat gout.

| Generic Name<br>*Brand Name* | Side Effects | Warnings | Dosing | Notes |
|---|---|---|---|---|
| **Allopurinol**<br>*Lopurin,*<br>*Zyloprim*<br>tablet (℞) | Stomach upset, headache, diarrhea, gastritis, fever, nausea, and vomiting. | May cause drowsiness. Contact a physician at the first sign of a rash, painful urination, or bloody urine. | Take with food or milk. Drink at least 10 to 12 full (8-oz.) glasses of fluids a day. Avoid large doses of Vitamin C. | May also be prescribed for managing uric acid blood levels secondary to leukemia and other malignancies. Also used to manage some types of kidney stones. |

**ACTION** Gout agents work either by reducing the formation of uric acid in the body or by decreasing the inflammatory response to uric acid.

**INDICATION** Used to treat gout.

| Generic Name<br>*Brand Name* | Side Effects | Warnings | Dosing | Notes |
|---|---|---|---|---|
| **Colchicine**<br>*Colchicine*<br>tablet (℞) | Vomiting, nausea, diarrhea, abdominal pain. | Stop taking at the first sign of stomach pain, nausea, vomiting or diarrhea. Contact a physician if rash, sore throat, unusual bleeding or bruising, weakness, fever, or tingling occurs. | Stop taking when gout pain is relieved. | May also be prescribed to prevent acute attacks of gout. |
| **Colchicine, Probenecid**<br>*ColBenemid*<br>tablet (℞) | Vomiting, nausea, diarrhea, abdominal pain, loss of appetite. | Stop taking at the first sign of stomach pain, nausea, vomiting or diarrhea. Contact a physician if rash, sore throat, unusual bleeding or bruising, weakness, fever, or tingling occurs. | Stop taking when gout pain is relieved. Take with food or antacids. Drink at least 6 to 8 full (8-oz.) glasses of fluids daily. Avoid the use of aspirin or aspirin-like products because they can block the effect of probenecid. | May also be prescribed to prevent acute attacks of gout. |
| **Probenecid**<br>*Benemid*<br>tablet (℞) | Nausea, vomiting, loss of appetite. | Avoid the use of aspirin or aspirin-like products because they can block the effect of probenecid. | Take with food or antacids. Drink at least 6 to 8 full (8-oz.) glasses of fluids daily. | May also be prescribed in conjunction with some antibiotics to make the antibiotic more effective in treating an infection. |

**ACTION** Gout agents work either by reducing the formation of uric acid in the body or by decreasing the inflammatory response to uric acid.

**INDICATION** Used to treat gout.

| Generic Name<br>*Brand Name* | Side Effects | Warnings | Dosing | Notes |
|---|---|---|---|---|
| **Sulfinpyrazone**<br>*Anturane* tablet,<br>capsule (℞) | Stomach upset,<br>nausea, vomiting,<br>loss of appetite,<br>painful urination. | Avoid the use of<br>aspirin or aspirin-<br>like products<br>because they can<br>block the effect of<br>Sulfinpyrazone. | Take with food,<br>milk or antacids.<br>Drink at least 10<br>to 12 full (8-oz.)<br>glasses of fluids<br>daily. | Used to treat<br>chronic gouty<br>arthritis. |

# Narcotic Agonist–Antagonist Analgesics

**ACTION** Work by competing with other substances at $\mu$ receptors that mediate pain. They are potent analgesics with a lower abuse potential than pure narcotic agonists.

**INDICATION** Used as a pain reliever and analgesic.

| Generic Name<br>*Brand Name* | Side Effects | Warnings | Dosing | Notes |
|---|---|---|---|---|
| **Butorphanol**<br>**Tartrate**<br>*Stadol* nasal<br>spray (℞, C-IV) | Drowsiness, diz-<br>ziness, nausea,<br>vomiting, consti-<br>pation, appetite<br>loss, nasal<br>congestion,<br>cough. | Avoid alcohol and<br>other drowsiness-<br>causing drugs.<br>This medication<br>has abuse poten-<br>tial. Dependence<br>may develop on<br>repeated use. | Clean nasal<br>passages before<br>using. May take<br>1 to 2 hours<br>to work. | Used for<br>treatment of<br>migraine<br>headaches. |
| **Pentazocine,**<br>**Naloxone HCl**<br>*Talwin NX* tablet<br>(℞, C-IV) | Drowsiness, diz-<br>ziness, skin rash,<br>difficult breath-<br>ing, confusion. | Avoid alcohol<br>and drowsiness-<br>causing drugs.<br>Contact physician<br>if rash, disorien-<br>tation or confu-<br>sion occurs. | Do not take in<br>anticipation of<br>pain, only for<br>existing pain. | |

# Narcotic Analgesics

**ACTION** Narcotic analgesics work by dulling the pain perception center in the brain. They can also affect other body systems at higher doses to produce respiratory and circulatory depression, shock, or apnea. Some narcotics are natural (e.g., opium, codeine, and morphine) and some are synthetic (e.g., opioids). Potency, addictive ability, and side effects vary among the narcotic analgesics. Tolerance to the analgesic effect is a sign of dependence.

**INDICATION** Used to relieve moderate to severe pain. Used to prepare patients for anesthesia and surgery. Always use caution when performing tasks requiring alertness.

| Generic Name<br>*Brand Name* | Side Effects | Warnings | Dosing | Notes |
|---|---|---|---|---|
| **Codeine**<br>*Codeine Sulfate*<br>tablet (℞, C-II) | Drowsiness, dizziness, blurred vision, nausea, vomiting, constipation, sweating. | Avoid alcohol and other drowsiness-causing drugs that can intensify overall sedation. | Take with food. | Used in low doses in combination with other medications as a cough suppressant. |
| **Hydromorphone**<br>*Dilaudid* tablet<br>(℞, C-II) | Drowsiness, dizziness, blurred vision, nausea, vomiting, constipation, sweating. | Avoid alcohol and other drowsiness-causing drugs that can intensify overall sedation. | Take with food. | |
| **Levorphanol Tartrate**<br>*Levo-Dromoran*<br>tablet (℞, C-II) | Drowsiness, dizziness, blurred vision, nausea, vomiting, constipation, sweating. | Avoid alcohol and other drowsiness-causing drugs that can intensify overall sedation. | Take with food. | |
| **Meperidine**<br>*Demerol* tablet,<br>syrup (℞, C-II) | Drowsiness, dizziness, blurred vision, nausea, vomiting, constipation, sweating. | Avoid alcohol and other drowsiness-causing drugs that can intensify overall sedation. | Take with food. | |
| **Methadone**<br>*Dolophine* tablet<br>(℞, C-II) | Drowsiness, dizziness, blurred vision, nausea, vomiting, constipation, sweating. | Avoid alcohol and other drowsiness-causing drugs that can intensify overall sedation. | Take with food. | Used for detoxification and treatment of narcotic addiction. |

**ACTION** Narcotic analgesics work by dulling the pain perception center in the brain. They can also affect other body systems at higher doses to produce respiratory and circulatory depression, shock, or apnea. Some narcotics are natural (e.g., opium, codeine, and morphine) and some are synthetic (e.g., opioids). Potency, addictive ability, and side effects vary among the narcotic analgesics. Tolerance to the analgesic effect is a sign of dependence.

**INDICATION** Used to relieve moderate to severe pain. Used to prepare patients for anesthesia and surgery. Always use caution when performing tasks requiring alertness.

| Generic Name<br>*Brand Name* | Side Effects | Warnings | Dosing | Notes |
|---|---|---|---|---|
| **Morphine Sulfate**<br>Morphine Sulfate<br>  tablet (℞, C-II)<br>*MS Contin,*<br>*Roxanol SR -*<br>  controlled release<br>  tablet (℞, C-II) | Drowsiness, dizziness, blurred vision, nausea, vomiting, constipation, sweating. | Avoid alcohol and other drowsiness-causing drugs that can intensify overall sedation. | Take with food. | Do not crush or chew controlled-release tablets. |
| **Opium**<br>*Opium Tincture*<br>  (℞, C-II)<br>*Paregoric*<br>  Liquid (℞, C-III) | Drowsiness, dizziness, blurred vision, nausea, vomiting, constipation, sweating. | Avoid alcohol and other drowsiness-causing drugs that can intensify overall sedation. | Take with food. | Used for its antidiarrheal effect. |
| **Oxycodone**<br>*Roxicodone* tablet<br>  (℞, C-II) | Drowsiness, dizziness, blurred vision, nausea, vomiting, constipation, sweating. | Avoid alcohol and other drowsiness-causing drugs that can intensify overall sedation. | Take with food. | |
| **Propoxyphene**<br>  **HCl**<br>*Darvon,*<br>*Dolene*<br>  capsule (℞, C-III) | Drowsiness, dizziness, blurred vision, nausea, vomiting, constipation, sweating. | Avoid alcohol and other drowsiness-causing drugs that can intensify overall sedation. | Take with food. | |
| **Propoxyphene**<br>  **Napsylate**<br>*Darvon-N*<br>  tablet (℞, C-III) | Drowsiness, dizziness, blurred vision, nausea, vomiting, constipation, sweating. | Avoid alcohol and other drowsiness-causing drugs that can intensify overall sedation. | Take with food. | |

## Narcotic Analgesic Combinations

**ACTION** Narcotic analgesics work by dulling the pain perception center in the brain. They can also affect other body systems at higher doses.

**INDICATION** Used to relieve moderate to severe pain. Narcotic analgesics are combined with other medications to either enhance the analgesic effect of the medication or to reduce side effects. It is important to consider the additional use of aspirin or acetaminophen, either singly or in other medication, combinations with what may be received in one of these products.

| Generic Name<br>*Brand Name* | Side Effects | Warnings | Dosing | Notes |
|---|---|---|---|---|
| **Codeine,**<br>**Acetaminophen**<br>*Tylenol w/Codeine*<br>tablet, elixir<br>(℞, C-III)<br>*Phenaphen*<br>*w/Codeine*<br>capsule (℞, C-III) | Drowsiness, dizziness, blurred vision, nausea, vomiting, constipation, sweating. | Avoid alcohol and other drowsiness-causing drugs that can intensify overall sedation. | Take with food. | |
| **Codeine,**<br>**Acetaminophen,**<br>**Butalbital,**<br>**Caffeine**<br>*Fioricet*<br>*w/Codeine*<br>capsule (℞, C-III) | Drowsiness, dizziness, blurred vision, nausea, vomiting, constipation, sweating. | Avoid alcohol and other drowsiness-causing drugs that can intensify overall sedation. | Take with food. | Caffeine may cause insomnia, excitement, nervousness, and tachycardia. |
| **Codeine, Aspirin**<br>*Empirin w/Codeine*<br>tablet (℞, C-III) | Drowsiness, dizziness, blurred vision, nausea, vomiting, constipation, sweating. | Avoid alcohol and other drowsiness-causing drugs that can intensify overall sedation. | Take with food. | |
| **Codeine, Aspirin,**<br>**Butalbital,**<br>**Caffeine**<br>*Fiorinal w/Codeine*<br>capsule (℞, C-III) | Drowsiness, dizziness, blurred vision, nausea, vomiting, constipation, sweating. | Avoid alcohol and other drowsiness-causing drugs that can intensify overall sedation. | Take with food. | Caffeine may cause insomnia, excitement, nervousness, and tachycardia. |
| **Hydrocodone**<br>**Bitartrate,**<br>**Acetaminophen**<br>*Lortab, Anesia,*<br>*Vicodin, Lorcet,*<br>*Hydocet* tablet and<br>capsule (℞, C-III) | Drowsiness, dizziness, blurred vision, nausea, vomiting, constipation, sweating. | Avoid alcohol and other drowsiness-causing drugs that can intensify overall sedation. | Take with food. | There are numerous other brand names in a variety of strengths. |

Analgesics

**ACTION** Narcotic analgesics work by dulling the pain perception center in the brain. They can also affect other body systems at higher doses.

**INDICATION** Used to relieve moderate to severe pain. Narcotic analgesics are combined with other medications to either enhance the analgesic effect of the medication or to reduce side effects. It is important to consider the additional use of aspirin or acetaminophen, either singly or in other medication, combinations with what may be received in one of these products.

| Generic Name<br>*Brand Name* | Side Effects | Warnings | Dosing | Notes |
|---|---|---|---|---|
| **Dihydrocodone Bitartrate, Aspirin**<br>*Lortab ASA, Azdone*<br>tablet (℞, C-III) | Drowsiness, dizziness, blurred vision, nausea, vomiting, constipation, sweating. | Avoid alcohol and other drowsiness-causing drugs that can intensify overall sedation. | Take with food. | |
| **Dihydrocodone Bitartrate, Aspirin, Caffeine**<br>*Synalgos DC*<br>capsule (℞, C-III) | Drowsiness, dizziness, blurred vision, nausea, vomiting, constipation, sweating. | Avoid alcohol and other drowsiness-causing drugs that can intensify overall sedation. | Take with food. | Caffeine may cause insomnia, excitement, nervousness, and tachycardia. |
| **Oxycodone Bitartrate, Acetaminophen**<br>*Percocet, Roxicet*<br>tablet (℞, C-II)<br>*Tylox, Roxilox*<br>capsule (℞, C-II) | Drowsiness, dizziness, blurred vision, nausea, vomiting, constipation, sweating. | Avoid alcohol and other drowsiness-causing drugs that can intensify overall sedation. | Take with food. | |
| **Oxycodone Bitartrate, Aspirin**<br>*Percodan, Roxiprin*<br>tablet (℞, C-II) | Drowsiness, dizziness, blurred vision, nausea, vomiting, constipation, sweating. | Avoid alcohol and other drowsiness-causing drugs that can intensify overall sedation. | Take with food. | |
| **Meperidine, Promethazine**<br>*Mepergan Fortis*<br>capsule (℞, C-II) | Drowsiness, dizziness, blurred vision, nausea, vomiting, constipation, sweating. | Avoid alcohol and other drowsiness-causing drugs that can intensify overall sedation. | Take with food. | Promethazine is used for its additional sedative effect and to reduce the effects of nausea and vomiting. |

**ACTION** Narcotic analgesics work by dulling the pain perception center in the brain. They can also affect other body systems at higher doses.

**INDICATION** Used to relieve moderate to severe pain. Narcotic analgesics are combined with other medications to either enhance the analgesic effect of the medication or to reduce side effects. It is important to consider the additional use of aspirin or acetaminophen, either singly or in other medication, combinations with what may be received in one of these products.

| Generic Name<br>*Brand Name* | Side Effects | Warnings | Dosing | Notes |
|---|---|---|---|---|
| **Propoxyphene HCl, Acetaminophen**<br>*Wygesic, Genagesic*<br>tablet (℞, C-IV) | Drowsiness, dizziness, blurred vision, nausea, vomiting, constipation, sweating. | Avoid alcohol and other drowsiness-causing drugs that can intensify overall sedation. | Take with food. | |
| **Propoxyphene Napsylate, Aspirin**<br>*Darvocet N, Propacet*<br>tablet (℞, C-IV) | Drowsiness, dizziness, blurred vision, nausea, vomiting, constipation, sweating. | Avoid alcohol and other drowsiness-causing drugs that can intensify overall sedation. | Take with food. | |
| **Propoxyphene HCl, Aspirin, Caffeine**<br>*Darvon Compound*<br>capsule (℞, C-IV) | Drowsiness, dizziness, blurred vision, nausea, vomiting, constipation, sweating. | Avoid alcohol and other drowsiness-causing drugs that can intensify overall sedation. | Take with food. | |

# Nonsteroidal Anti-Inflammatory Drugs (NSAIDs)

**ACTION** NSAIDs work by reducing inflammation (pain, swelling, redness, heat) and by inhibiting chemicals in the body that produce tissue irritation and cause inflammation.

**INDICATION** Used for pain, fever, anti-inflammatory effects, and arthritis pain relief. NSAIDs are also used for mild to moderate pain resulting from conditions such as headache, dental pain, athletic injury, menstrual cramps, flu, colds, and sore throats. They may also be prescribed for rheumatoid arthritis, sunburn, gouty arthritis, ankylosing spondylitis, bursitis, tendinitis, osteoarthritis, and migraine headaches.

| Generic Name<br>*Brand Name* | Side Effects | Warnings | Dosing | Notes |
|---|---|---|---|---|
| **Bromfenac Sodium**<br>Duract capsule (]) | Gastrointestinal effects, constipation, diarrhea, dyspepsia, flatulence, nausea, vomiting. | Avoid long-term use, which can increase the risk of hepatotoxicity. | Avoid taking the drug with food. | Not to be used for conditions such as osteoarthritis and rheumatoid arthritis. |
| **Diclofenac Potassium**<br>*Cataflam* tablet (℞) | Stomach upset, ulceration, drowsiness, dizziness, blurred vision, sensitivity to sunlight. | Avoid aspirin and alcoholic beverages, which can increase the risk for stomach upset and ulceration. | Take with food. | |
| **Diclofenac Sodium**<br>*Voltaren* delayed-release tablet (℞) | Stomach upset, ulceration, drowsiness, dizziness, blurred vision, sensitivity to sunlight. | Avoid aspirin and alcoholic beverages, which can increase the risk for stomach upset and ulceration. | Take with food. | Do not crush the tablet. |
| **Etodolac**<br>*Lodine* capsule, tablet (℞)<br>*Lodine XL* extended-release tablet (℞) | Stomach upset, ulceration, drowsiness, dizziness, blurred vision, sensitivity to sunlight. | Avoid aspirin and alcoholic beverages, which can increase the risk for stomach upset and ulceration. | Take with food. | Do not crush the extended-release tablet. |

**ACTION** NSAIDs work by reducing inflammation (pain, swelling, redness, heat) and by inhibiting chemicals in the body that produce tissue irritation and cause inflammation.

**INDICATION** Used for pain, fever, anti-inflammatory effects, and arthritis pain relief. NSAIDs are also used for mild to moderate pain resulting from conditions such as headache, dental pain, athletic injury, menstrual cramps, flu, colds, and sore throats. They may also be prescribed for rheumatoid arthritis, sunburn, gouty arthritis, ankylosing spondylitis, bursitis, tendinitis, osteoarthritis, and migraine headaches.

| Generic Name<br>*Brand Name* | Side Effects | Warnings | Dosing | Notes |
|---|---|---|---|---|
| **Fenoprofen Calcium**<br>*Nalfon* capsule, tablet (℞) | Stomach upset, ulceration, drowsiness, dizziness, blurred vision, sensitivity to sunlight. | Avoid aspirin and alcoholic beverages, which can increase the risk for stomach upset and ulceration. Advise a physician if fever, rash, joint pain, or decreased urination occur. | Take with food. | |
| **Flurbiprofen**<br>Ansaid tablet (℞) | Stomach upset, ulceration, drowsiness, dizziness, blurred vision, sensitivity to sunlight. | Avoid aspirin and alcoholic beverages, which can increase the risk for stomach upset and ulceration. | Take with food. | |
| **Ibuprofen**<br>*Advil, Motrin IB* tablets or caplet (OTC)<br>*Children's Motrin* Suspension (OTC)<br>*Motrin, Rufen* tablets (℞) | Stomach upset, ulceration, drowsiness, dizziness, blurred vision, sensitivity to sunlight. | Avoid aspirin and alcoholic beverages, which can increase the risk for stomach upset and ulceration. | Take with food. | OTC Use—Do not take for more than 3 days for fever or 10 days for pain. Do not take more than 1200 mg in 24 hours without consulting a physician. |

**ACTION** NSAIDs work by reducing inflammation (pain, swelling, redness, heat) and by inhibiting chemicals in the body that produce tissue irritation and cause inflammation.

**INDICATION** Used for pain, fever, anti-inflammatory effects, and arthritis pain relief. NSAIDs are also used for mild to moderate pain resulting from conditions such as headache, dental pain, athletic injury, menstrual cramps, flu, colds, and sore throats. They may also be prescribed for rheumatoid arthritis, sunburn, gouty arthritis, ankylosing spondylitis, bursitis, tendinitis, osteoarthritis, and migraine headaches.

| Generic Name<br>*Brand Name* | Side Effects | Warnings | Dosing | Notes |
|---|---|---|---|---|
| **Indomethacin**<br>*Indocin*<br>  capsules (℞)<br>*Indocin SR*<br>  sustained-release<br>  capsules (℞) | Headaches, stomach upset, ulceration, drowsiness, dizziness, blurred vision, sensitivity to sunlight. | Avoid aspirin and alcoholic beverages, which can increase the risk for stomach upset and ulceration. If severe CNS adverse reactions develop, contact a physician. | Take with food. | |
| **Ketoprofen**<br>*Actron, Orudis KT*<br>  tablets (OTC)<br>*Orudis*<br>  capsules (℞)<br>*Oruvail* time-<br>  release capsules<br>  (℞) | Stomach upset, ulceration, drowsiness, dizziness, blurred vision, sensitivity to sunlight. | Avoid aspirin and alcoholic beverages, which can increase the risk for stomach upset and ulceration. | Take with food. | OTC Use—Do not exceed 25 mg in a 4- to 6-hour period or 75 mg in 24 hours. |
| **Ketorolac**<br>  **Tromethamine**<br>*Toradol* tablet (℞) | Stomach upset, ulceration, drowsiness, dizziness, blurred vision, sensitivity to sunlight. | Avoid aspirin and alcoholic beverages, which can increase the risk for stomach upset and ulceration. Not to be used for more than 5 days. | Take with food. | Not for minor or chronic pain use. |

**ACTION** NSAIDs work by reducing inflammation (pain, swelling, redness, heat) and by inhibiting chemicals in the body that produce tissue irritation and cause inflammation.

**INDICATION** Used for pain, fever, anti-inflammatory effects, and arthritis pain relief. NSAIDs are also used for mild to moderate pain resulting from conditions such as headache, dental pain, athletic injury, menstrual cramps, flu, colds, and sore throats. They may also be prescribed for rheumatoid arthritis, sunburn, gouty arthritis, ankylosing spondylitis, bursitis, tendinitis, osteoarthritis, and migraine headaches.

| Generic Name<br>*Brand Name* | Side Effects | Warnings | Dosing | Notes |
|---|---|---|---|---|
| **Meclofenamate Sodium**<br>*Meclomen* capsule (℞) | Stomach upset, ulceration, drowsiness, dizziness, blurred vision, sensitivity to sunlight. | Avoid aspirin and alcoholic beverages, which can increase the risk for stomach upset and ulceration. If rash, diarrhea, or other digestive problems occur call a physician. | Take with food. | |
| **Mefenamic Acid**<br>*Ponstel* capsule (℞) | Stomach upset, ulceration, drowsiness, dizziness, blurred vision, sensitivity to sunlight. | Avoid aspirin and alcoholic beverages, which can increase the risk for stomach upset and ulceration. Not to be used for more than 1 week. If rash, diarrhea, or digestive problems occur call your physician. | Take with food. | |
| **Nabumetone**<br>*Relafen* tablet (℞) | Stomach upset, ulceration, drowsiness, dizziness, blurred vision, sensitivity to sunlight. | Avoid aspirin and alcoholic beverages. | Take with food. | |

Analgesics

**ACTION** NSAIDs work by reducing inflammation (pain, swelling, redness, heat) and by inhibiting chemicals in the body that produce tissue irritation and cause inflammation.

**INDICATION** Used for pain, fever, anti-inflammatory effects, and arthritis pain relief. NSAIDs are also used for mild to moderate pain resulting from conditions such as headache, dental pain, athletic injury, menstrual cramps, flu, colds, and sore throats. They may also be prescribed for rheumatoid arthritis, sunburn, gouty arthritis, ankylosing spondylitis, bursitis, tendinitis, osteoarthritis, and migraine headaches.

| Generic Name<br>*Brand Name* | Side Effects | Warnings | Dosing | Notes |
|---|---|---|---|---|
| **Naproxen**<br>*Naprosyn* tablet (℞)<br>*EC-Naprosyn*<br>  delayed-release<br>  tablets (℞) | Stomach upset, ulceration, drowsiness, dizziness, blurred vision, sensitivity to sunlight. | Avoid aspirin and alcoholic beverages, which can increase the risk for stomach upset and ulceration. | Take with food. | Do not crush delayed-release tablets. |
| **Naproxen Sodium**<br>*Aleve* tablets or<br>  caplet (OTC)<br>*Anaprox,*<br>*Anaprox DS*<br>  tablets (℞) | Stomach upset, ulceration, drowsiness, dizziness, blurred vision, sensitivity to sunlight. | Avoid aspirin and alcoholic beverages, which can increase the risk for stomach upset and ulceration. | Take with food. | OTC Use—Do not take more than 3 days for fever or 10 days for pain, and do not take more than 660 mg in 24 hours. |
| **Oxaprozin**<br>*Daypro* caplet (℞) | Stomach upset, ulceration, drowsiness, dizziness, blurred vision, sensitivity to sunlight. | Avoid aspirin and alcoholic beverages, which can increase the risk for stomach upset and ulceration. | Take with food. | |
| **Piroxicam**<br>*Feldene*<br>  capsule (℞) | Stomach upset, ulceration, drowsiness, dizziness, blurred vision, sensitivity to sunlight. | Avoid aspirin and alcoholic beverages, which can increase the risk for stomach upset and ulceration. Not to be used for more than 5 days. | Take with food. | |

**ACTION** NSAIDs work by reducing inflammation (pain, swelling, redness, heat) and by inhibiting chemicals in the body that produce tissue irritation and cause inflammation.

**INDICATION** Used for pain, fever, anti-inflammatory effects, and arthritis pain relief. NSAIDs are also used for mild to moderate pain resulting from conditions such as headache, dental pain, athletic injury, menstrual cramps, flu, colds, and sore throats. They may also be prescribed for rheumatoid arthritis, sunburn, gouty arthritis, ankylosing spondylitis, bursitis, tendinitis, osteoarthritis, and migraine headaches.

| Generic Name<br>*Brand Name* | Side Effects | Warnings | Dosing | Notes |
|---|---|---|---|---|
| **Sulindac**<br>*Clinoril* tablet (℞) | Stomach upset, ulceration, drowsiness, dizziness, blurred vision, sensitivity to sunlight. | Avoid aspirin and alcoholic beverages, which can increase the risk for stomach upset and ulceration. If unexplained fever or other allergic reactions occur, stop using and contact a physician. | Take with food. | |
| **Tolmetin Sodium**<br>*Tolectin* capsule (℞)<br>*Tolectin DS* tablet (℞) | Stomach upset, ulceration, drowsiness, dizziness, blurred vision, sensitivity to sunlight. | Avoid aspirin and alcoholic beverages, which can increase the risk for stomach upset and ulceration. | Take with food. | |

# Migraine Agents

**ACTION** Agents for migraine treatment generally work either by reducing blood flow in the cranial arteries or by inhibiting a chemical mediator that may cause vascular headaches.

**INDICATION** Used to treat migraines (vascular headaches).

| Generic Name<br>*Brand Name* | Side Effects | Warnings | Dosing | Notes |
|---|---|---|---|---|
| **Ergotamine Tartrate**<br>*Ergomar, Ergostat*<br>sublingual tablet (℞)<br>*Medihaler Ergotamine*<br>aerosol (℞) | Muscle pain, nausea, vomiting, localized edema, itching. | Do not exceed the recommended daily dose. Contact physician if heart rate changes; nausea, vomiting, numbness, or tingling in fingers or toes occurs; or there is a weakness of extremities. | Tablets should be dissolved under the tongue. Initiate therapy at first sign of symptoms. | Also used for cluster headaches. |
| **Ergotamine Tartrate, Caffeine**<br>*Cafergot, Ercaf, Wigraine*<br>tablet (℞)<br>*Cafergot, Wigraine*<br>rectal suppository (℞) | Muscle pain, nausea, vomiting, localized edema, itching. | Do not exceed the recommended daily dose. Contact physician if heart rate changes; nausea, vomiting, numbness, or tingling in fingers or toes occurs; or there is a weakness of extremities. | Tablets should be dissolved under the tongue. Initiate therapy at first sign of symptoms. | Also used for cluster headaches. Caffeine can constrict blood vessels and may enhance the absorption of ergotamine. |
| **Isometheptene Mucate, Dichloralphenazone, Acetaminophen**<br>*Isocom, Midrin*<br>capsule (℞) | Transient dizziness, rash, muscle pain, nausea, vomiting, localized edema, itching. | Do not exceed the recommended daily dose. May cause drowsiness. | Is important to consider the additional use of acetaminophen in other products with what is in this medication (325 mg). Initiate therapy at first sign of symptoms. | Acetaminophen is used for pain relief and Dichloralphenazone is used for sedation. |

**ACTION** Agents for migraine treatment generally work either by reducing blood flow in the cranial arteries or by inhibiting a chemical mediator that may cause vascular headaches.

**INDICATION** Used to treat migraines (vascular headaches).

| Generic Name<br>*Brand Name* | Side Effects | Warnings | Dosing | Notes |
|---|---|---|---|---|
| **Methysergide Maleate**<br>*Sansert*<br>tablet (R) | Insomnia, dizziness, weakness, edema, facial flush, diarrhea, constipation. | Notify a physician if cold or numb hands and feet, leg cramps, chest pain, painful urination, or shortness of breath. May also cause drowsiness. | Take with food or milk to avoid GI upset. | This medication is used only to prevent migraine headaches. It is not used to treat a migraine once it has started. |
| **Sumatriptan Succinate**<br>*Imitrex* tablet, injection (R) | Drowsiness, dizziness, tiredness, flushing, nausea. | Do not take more than 300 mg in 24 hours. Contact physician if shortness of breath, rash, or pain in chest or throat. | Tablets may be taken without regard to food. | Also used for preattack symptoms of migraine. |

Analgesics

# Salicylates

**ACTION** Salicylates lower elevated body temperatures (fever) by vasodilation of peripheral blood vessels, which enhances body heat loss. Salicylates act as analgesic and anti-inflammatory agents through inhibition of certain prostaglandins.

**INDICATION** For use of mild and moderate pain, fever, and inflammatory conditions associated with osteoarthritis, rheumatoid arthritis, or rheumatic fever. Do not use in children or teenagers for chickenpox or flu symptoms.

| Generic Name<br>*Brand Name* | Side Effects | Warnings | Dosing | Notes |
|---|---|---|---|---|
| **Aspirin (ASA)**<br>*Bayer Aspirin,*<br>*Empirin* tablet (OTC)<br>*Ecotrin* enteric<br>  coated tablet<br>  (OTC)<br>*ZORprin*<br>  controlled-release<br>  tablet (℞)<br>*Aspergum* gum<br>  tablet (OTC)<br>*Bayer Children's*<br>  chewable tablet<br>  (OTC)<br>*Aspirin*<br>  suppository (OTC) | Nausea, dyspepsia, heartburn, epigastric discomfort, GI bleeding. | Alcohol increases the risk of GI ulceration. | Take with food or after meals to avoid GI upset. Take with full glass of water to avoid the risk of the medication lodging in the esophagus. Do not crush enteric coated tablet. | Used to reduce the risk of myocardial infarctions (MI) and stroke in patients with a previous history of MI and stroke. Aspirin is commonly found in combination with other medications such as cough and cold or analgesics. Do not exceed 4 grams in 24 hours. |
| **Buffered Aspirin**<br>*Bufferin, Ascriptin*<br>  *A/D* tablet (OTC)<br>*Alka-Seltzer with*<br>  *Aspirin* effervescent<br>  tablet (OTC) | Nausea, dyspepsia, heartburn, epigastric discomfort, GI bleeding. | Alcohol increases the risk of GI ulceration. | Take with food or after meals to avoid GI upset. Take with full glass of water to avoid the risk of the medication's lodging in the esophagus. | These products contain small amounts of antacids (calcium carbonate, magnesium hydroxide, aluminum hydroxide, and others) to decrease GI irritation or to increase the absorption. |

**ACTION** Salicylates lower elevated body temperatures (fever) by vasodilation of peripheral blood vessels, which enhances body heat loss. Salicylates act as analgesic and anti-inflammatory agents through inhibition of certain prostaglandins.

**INDICATION** For use of mild and moderate pain, fever, and inflammatory conditions associated with osteoarthritis, rheumatoid arthritis, or rheumatic fever. Do not use in children or teenagers for chickenpox or flu symptoms.

| Generic Name<br>*Brand Name* | Side Effects | Warnings | Dosing | Notes |
|---|---|---|---|---|
| **Choline Salicylate**<br>*Arthropan* liquid<br>(OTC) | Nausea, dyspepsia, heartburn, epigastric discomfort, GI bleeding. | Alcohol increases the risk of GI ulceration. | Take with food or after meals to avoid GI upset. | Has fewer GI side effects than aspirin. |
| **Choline Salicylate, Magnesium Salicylate**<br>*Trilisate*<br>tablet (℞) | Nausea, dyspepsia, heartburn, epigastric discomfort, GI bleeding. | Alcohol increases the risk of GI ulceration. | Take with food or after meals to avoid GI upset. Take with full glass of water to avoid the risk of the medication's lodging in the esophagus. | |
| **Diflunisal**<br>*Dolobid* tablet (℞) | Nausea, dyspepsia, GI pain, diarrhea, vomiting, constipation, headache, insomnia, GI bleeding. | Do not take with aspirin or acetaminophen. | Take with food or after meals to avoid GI upset. Do not crush or chew tablet. | |
| **Magnesium Salicylate**<br>*Doan's* caplet (OTC)<br>*Magan, Mobidin*<br>tablet (℞) | Nausea, dyspepsia, heartburn, epigastric discomfort, GI bleeding. | Alcohol increases the risk of GI ulceration. | Take with food or after meals to avoid GI upset. Take with full glass of water to avoid the risk of the medication's lodging in the esophagus. | As a sodium-free salicylate, may have lower incidence of GI upset than aspirin. |

**ACTION** Salicylates lower elevated body temperatures (fever) by vasodilation of peripheral blood vessels, which enhances body heat loss. Salicylates act as analgesic and anti-inflammatory agents through inhibition of certain prostaglandins.

**INDICATION** For use of mild and moderate pain, fever, and inflammatory conditions associated with osteoarthritis, rheumatoid arthritis, or rheumatic fever. Do not use in children or teenagers for chickenpox or flu symptoms.

| Generic Name<br>Brand Name | Side Effects | Warnings | Dosing | Notes |
|---|---|---|---|---|
| **Salsalate**<br>*Disalcid, Amigesic,*<br>*Salflex* capsule,<br>tablet (R) | Nausea, dyspepsia, heartburn, epigastric discomfort, GI bleeding. | Alcohol increases the risk of GI ulceration. | Take with food or after meals to avoid GI upset. Take with full glass of water to avoid the risk of the medication's lodging in the esophagus. | |

## Nonnarcotic Analgesic Combinations

There is a tremendous number of combinations of nonnarcotic analgesics with other products. They are combined with sedatives, caffeine, antacids, and diuretics. More information is found under individual drugs elsewhere in the book

**BANNED SUBSTANCES** NCAA and/or USOC may list some of these substances as banned for athletes to use.

| Brand Name | Nonnarcotic | Sedatives/Stimulant | Other |
|---|---|---|---|
| *Anacin* (OTC) | Aspirin | Caffeine | |
| *Aspirin Free*<br>*Excedrin* (OTC) | Acetaminophen | Caffeine | |
| *Axotal* (R) | Aspirin | Caffeine, Butalbital | |
| *B-A-C* (R) | Aspirin | Caffeine, Butalbital | |
| *Bancap* (R) | Acetaminophen | Butalbital | |
| *BC Powder* (OTC) | Aspirin, Salicylamide | | Sodium Aminobenzoate |
| *Cope* (OTC) | Aspirin | Caffeine | Magnesium and Aluminum Hydroxide |
| *Equagesic* (R, C-IV) | Aspirin | Meprobamate | |

There is a tremendous number of combinations of nonnarcotic analgesics with other products. They are combined with sedatives, caffeine, antacids, and diuretics. More information is found under individual drugs elsewhere in the book

**BANNED SUBSTANCES** NCAA and/or USOC may list some of these substances as banned for athletes to use.

| Brand Name | Nonnarcotic | Sedatives/Stimulant | Other |
|---|---|---|---|
| Esgic (℞) | Acetaminophen | Caffeine, Butalbital | |
| Excedrin (OTC) | Acetaminophen, Aspirin | Caffeine | |
| Extra Strength Tylenol Headache Plus (OTC) | Acetaminophen | | Calcium Carbonate |
| Femcet (℞) | Acetaminophen | Caffeine, Butalbital | |
| Fioricet (℞) | Acetaminophen | Caffeine, Butalbital | |
| Fiorinal (℞, C-III) | Aspirin | Caffeine, Butalbital | |
| Isollyl (℞, C-III) | Aspirin | Caffeine, Butalbital | |
| Magsal (℞) | Magnesium Salicylate | Phenyltoloxamine Citrate | |
| Medigesic (℞) | Acetaminophen | Caffeine, Butalbital | |
| Micrainin (℞, C-IV) | Aspirin | Meprobamate | |
| Mobigesic (OTC) | Magnesium Salicylate | Phenyltoloxamine Citrate | |
| Momentum (OTC) | Aspirin | Phenyltoloxamine Citrate | |
| Pabalate Enteric Coated (OTC) | Sodium Salicylate | | Sodium Aminobenzoate |
| Phrenilin (℞) | Acetaminophen | Butalbital | |
| Premsyn PMS (OTC) | Acetaminophen | Pyrilamine Maleate | Pamabrom |
| SedAcetaminophen-10 (℞) | Acetaminophen | Butalbital | |
| Vanquish (OTC) | Acetaminophen, Aspirin | Caffeine | Magnesium and Aluminum Hydroxide |

# Respiratory Agents

## Antihistamines

**ACTION** Antihistamines work by counteracting the chemical released by the body during an allergic reaction (histamine). Histamine causes itching, redness, watery eyes, runny nose, sneezing, and rashes.

**INDICATION** Used for seasonal and year-round allergies. Also used for mild to moderate rashes and insect bites and stings when there are no medical complications. Avoid "shotgun" therapy with combination products unless needed. Using a multiple-ingredient product when not necessary may increase the risk for side effects and drug interactions. Children and elderly may experience excitation, restlessness, and insomnia.

**BANNED SUBSTANCES** NCAA and/or USOC may list some of these substances as banned for athletes to use. Pseudoephedrine HCl may be banned in various situations.

| Generic Name<br>*Brand Name* | Side Effects | Warnings | Dosing | Notes |
|---|---|---|---|---|
| **Acrivastine,<br>Pseudoephedrine<br>HCl**<br>*Semprex-D* (℞) | Stomach upset, drowsiness, dizziness, dry mouth, sensitivity to the sun. | Care should be taken when performing tasks requiring alertness. | Can take with food if causes stomach upset. | Pseudoephedrine is a decongestant used in numerous other combination products. |
| **Astemizole**<br>*Hismanal* tablet (℞) | Drowsiness, dizziness, dry mouth, sensitivity to the sun. | Must be taken daily (not as needed). | Take on an empty stomach, 1 hour before or 2 hours after a meal. | |
| **Azatadine<br>Maleate**<br>*Optimine* tablet (℞) | Stomach upset, drowsiness, dizziness, dry mouth, sensitivity to the sun. | Care should be taken when performing tasks requiring alertness. | Can take with food if causes stomach upset. | |
| **Azelastine HCL**<br>*Astelin* spray (℞) | Bitter taste, headache, somnolence, nasal burning, pharyngitis, dry mouth, sneezing, nausea. | Do not use with other antihistamines. Avoid alcohol as it can further reduce alertness. | Blow nose to clear nostrils. | |

**ACTION** Antihistamines work by counteracting the chemical released by the body during an allergic reaction (histamine). Histamine causes itching, redness, watery eyes, runny nose, sneezing, and rashes.

**INDICATION** Used for seasonal and year-round allergies. Also used for mild to moderate rashes and insect bites and stings when there are no medical complications. Avoid "shotgun" therapy with combination products unless needed. Using a multiple-ingredient product when not necessary may increase the risk for side effects and drug interactions. Children and elderly may experience excitation, restlessness, and insomnia.

**BANNED SUBSTANCES** NCAA and/or USOC may list some of these substances as banned for athletes to use. Pseudoephedrine HCl may be banned in various situations.

| Generic Name<br>*Brand Name* | Side Effects | Warnings | Dosing | Notes |
|---|---|---|---|---|
| **Bromphenira-mine Maleate**<br>*Dimetane, Bromphen* tablet, elixir (OTC)<br>*Dimetane Exten-tabs* time-release tablets (OTC) | Stomach upset, drowsiness, dizziness, dry mouth, sensitivity to the sun. | Care should be taken when performing tasks requiring alertness. | Can take with food if causes stomach upset. | OTC Use—Do not take more than 24 mg in 24 hours. |
| **Carbinoxamine Maleate**<br>*Clistin* tablet (℞) | Stomach upset, drowsiness, dizziness, dry mouth, sensitivity to the sun. | Care should be taken when performing tasks requiring alertness. | Can take with food if causes stomach upset. | |
| **Cetirizine HCl**<br>*Zyrtec* tablet, syrup (℞) | Stomach upset, drowsiness, dizziness, dry mouth, sensitivity to the sun. | Care should be taken when performing tasks requiring alertness. | Can take with food if causes stomach upset. | OTC Use—Do not take more than 24 mg in 24 hours. |
| **Chlorphenira-mine Maleate**<br>*Chlor-Trimeton* tablet, syrup (OTC)<br>*Chlor-Trimeton Allergy, Efidac* time-release tablet (OTC)<br>*Teldrin* time-release capsule (OTC) | Stomach upset, drowsiness, dizziness, dry mouth, sensitivity to the sun. | Care should be taken when performing tasks requiring alertness. | Can take with food if causes stomach upset. | OTC Use—Do not take more than 24 mg in 24 hours. |

**ACTION** Antihistamines work by counteracting the chemical released by the body during an allergic reaction (histamine). Histamine causes itching, redness, watery eyes, runny nose, sneezing, and rashes.

**INDICATION** Used for seasonal and year-round allergies. Also used for mild to moderate rashes and insect bites and stings when there are no medical complications. Avoid "shotgun" therapy with combination products unless needed. Using a multiple-ingredient product when not necessary may increase the risk for side effects and drug interactions. Children and elderly may experience excitation, restlessness, and insomnia.

**BANNED SUBSTANCES** NCAA and/or USOC may list some of these substances as banned for athletes to use. Pseudoephedrine HCl may be banned in various situations.

| Generic Name<br>*Brand Name* | Side Effects | Warnings | Dosing | Notes |
|---|---|---|---|---|
| **Clemastine<br>Fumarate**<br>*Tavist-1* tablet<br>(OTC)<br>*Tavist* tablet,<br>syrup (℞) | Stomach upset,<br>drowsiness,<br>dizziness, dry<br>mouth, sensitiv-<br>ity to the sun. | Care should be<br>taken when<br>performing<br>tasks requiring<br>alertness. | Can take with<br>food if causes<br>stomach upset. | OTC Use—Do<br>not exceed 8 mg<br>in 24 hours. |
| **Cyproheptadine<br>HCl**<br>*Periactin* tablet,<br>syrup (℞) | Stomach upset,<br>drowsiness,<br>dizziness, dry<br>mouth, sensitiv-<br>ity to the sun. | Care should be<br>taken when<br>performing<br>tasks requiring<br>alertness. | Can take with<br>food if causes<br>stomach upset. | |
| **Dexchlorphenira-<br>mine Maleate**<br>*Polaramine*<br>tablet, syrup (℞)<br>*Polaramine,<br>Dexchlor* time-<br>release tablet (℞) | Stomach upset,<br>drowsiness,<br>dizziness, dry<br>mouth, sensitiv-<br>ity to the sun. | Care should be<br>taken when<br>performing<br>tasks requiring<br>alertness. | Can take with<br>food if causes<br>stomach upset. | |
| **Diphenhydramine<br>Maleate**<br>*Benadryl*<br>tablet, capsule,<br>elixir, liquid,<br>syrup (OTC) | Stomach upset,<br>drowsiness,<br>dizziness, dry<br>mouth, sensitiv-<br>ity to the sun. | Care should be<br>taken when<br>performing<br>tasks requiring<br>alertness. | Can take with<br>food if causes<br>stomach upset. | This medication<br>is also used for<br>sleeplessness, to<br>prevent motion<br>sickness, and for<br>parkinsonism.<br>OTC Use—Do<br>not take more<br>than 300 mg in<br>24 hours. |

Respiratory

**ACTION** Antihistamines work by counteracting the chemical released by the body during an allergic reaction (histamine). Histamine causes itching, redness, watery eyes, runny nose, sneezing, and rashes.

**INDICATION** Used for seasonal and year-round allergies. Also used for mild to moderate rashes and insect bites and stings when there are no medical complications. Avoid "shotgun" therapy with combination products unless needed. Using a multiple-ingredient product when not necessary may increase the risk for side effects and drug interactions. Children and elderly may experience excitation, restlessness, and insomnia.

**BANNED SUBSTANCES** NCAA and/or USOC may list some of these substances as banned for athletes to use. Pseudoephedrine HCl may be banned in various situations.

| Generic Name<br>*Brand Name* | Side Effects | Warnings | Dosing | Notes |
|---|---|---|---|---|
| **Fexofenadine HCl**<br>*Allegra* capsule<br>(℞) | Stomach upset, drowsiness, dizziness, dry mouth, sensitivity to the sun. | Care should be taken when performing tasks requiring alertness. | Can take with food if causes stomach upset. | |
| **Loratadine**<br>*Claritin* tablet<br>(℞)<br>*Claritin RediTabs*<br>(℞) | Headache, somnolence, fatigue, dry mouth, dizziness, increased sweating, thirst, sensitivity to the sun. | Care should be taken when performing tasks requiring alertness. | Can take regardless of food. | RediTabs are to be dissolved under the tongue. |
| **Methdilazine HCl**<br>*Tacaryl* tablet, syrup (℞) | Stomach upset, drowsiness, dizziness, dry mouth, sensitivity to the sun. | Care should be taken when performing tasks requiring alertness. | Can take with food if causes stomach upset. | |
| **Phenindamine Tartrate**<br>*Nolahist* tablet<br>(OTC) | Stomach upset, drowsiness, dizziness, dry mouth, sensitivity to the sun. | Care should be taken when performing tasks requiring alertness. | Can take with food if causes stomach upset. | OTC Use—Do not take more than 150 mg in 24 hours. |

**ACTION** Antihistamines work by counteracting the chemical released by the body during an allergic reaction (histamine). Histamine causes itching, redness, watery eyes, runny nose, sneezing, and rashes.

**INDICATION** Used for seasonal and year-round allergies. Also used for mild to moderate rashes and insect bites and stings when there are no medical complications. Avoid "shotgun" therapy with combination products unless needed. Using a multiple-ingredient product when not necessary may increase the risk for side effects and drug interactions. Children and elderly may experience excitation, restlessness, and insomnia.

**BANNED SUBSTANCES** NCAA and/or USOC may list some of these substances as banned for athletes to use. Pseudoephedrine HCl may be banned in various situations.

| Generic Name  <br>*Brand Name* | Side Effects | Warnings | Dosing | Notes |
|---|---|---|---|---|
| **Promethazine HCl** <br>*Phenergan* <br> tablet, syrup, <br> suppository (℞) | Stomach upset, drowsiness, dizziness, dry mouth. Report any involuntary muscle movements or unusual sensitivity to sunlight. | Care should be taken when performing tasks requiring alertness. | Can take with food if causes stomach upset. | Used to treat motion sickness, nausea and vomiting, and sleeplessness. Also used in combination with pain medications to control pain. |
| **Pyrilamine Maleate, Pheniramine Maleate, Phenyltoloxamine Citrate** <br>*Poly-Histine* <br> elixir (OTC) | Stomach upset, drowsiness, dizziness, dry mouth, sensitivity to the sun. | Care should be taken when performing tasks requiring alertness. | Can take with food if causes stomach upset. | Combination of three different antihistamines. |
| **Terfenadine** <br>*Seldane* tablet <br> (℞) | Stomach upset, drowsiness, dizziness, dry mouth, sensitivity to the sun. | Care should be taken when performing tasks requiring alertness. | Can take with food if causes stomach upset. | Should not be taken while taking some other prescription medications. |
| **Trimeprazine** <br>*Temaril* tablet, <br> spansule, syrup <br> (℞) | Stomach upset, drowsiness, dizziness, dry mouth, sensitivity to the sun. | Care should be taken when performing tasks requiring alertness. | Can take with food if causes stomach upset. | |

**ACTION** Antihistamines work by counteracting the chemical released by the body during an allergic reaction (histamine). Histamine causes itching, redness, watery eyes, runny nose, sneezing, and rashes.

**INDICATION** Used for seasonal and year-round allergies. Also used for mild to moderate rashes and insect bites and stings when there are no medical complications. Avoid "shotgun" therapy with combination products unless needed. Using a multiple-ingredient product when not necessary may increase the risk for side effects and drug interactions. Children and elderly may experience excitation, restlessness, and insomnia.

**BANNED SUBSTANCES** NCAA and/or USOC may list some of these substances as banned for athletes to use. Pseudoephedrine HCl may be banned in various situations.

| Generic Name<br>*Brand Name* | Side Effects | Warnings | Dosing | Notes |
|---|---|---|---|---|
| **Tripelennamine HCl**<br>*PBZ, Pelamine*<br>tablet, elixir (℞)<br>*PBZ-SR*<br>sustained-release<br>tablet (℞) | Stomach upset, drowsiness, dizziness, dry mouth, sensitivity to the sun. | Care should be taken when performing tasks requiring alertness. | Can take with food if causes stomach upset. | |
| **Triprolidine HCl**<br>*Myidil* syrup (℞) | Stomach upset, drowsiness, dizziness, dry mouth, sensitivity to the sun. | Care should be taken when performing tasks requiring alertness. | Can take with food if causes stomach upset. | |

## Antitussives

**ACTION** Antitussives suppress the "cough center" of the brain. Coughing is a normal protective reflex that helps clear mucus and other irritants from the throat and lungs. A productive cough (mucus is coughed up) should not be suppressed. However, a dry nonproductive cough should be treated.

**INDICATION** Used to suppress cough due to irritation of the respiratory tract. **Codeine** and **Hydrocodone Bitartrate** are also used as cough suppressants at a lower dose than required for pain (see Narcotic Analgesics). Avoid "shotgun" therapy with combination products unless needed. Using a multiple-ingredient product when not necessary may increase the risk for side effects and drug interactions.

| Generic Name<br>*Brand Name* | Side Effects | Warnings | Dosing | Notes |
|---|---|---|---|---|
| **Dextromoth-orphan HBr**<br>*Benylin DM,*<br>*Robitussin*<br>*Pediatric* syrup<br>(OTC)<br>*Hold, Sucrets Cough*<br>*Control* lozenges<br>(OTC)<br>*Delsym* sustained<br>action liquid (OTC) | Constipation,<br>nausea, stomach<br>upset, sedation,<br>and itching. | Do not take for<br>chronic cough<br>associated<br>with smoking,<br>asthma,or<br>emphysema. | | OTC Use—If<br>cough continues<br>beyond 7 to 10<br>days, see a<br>doctor. |
| **Diphenhydra-mine HCl**<br>*Benylin Cough*<br>syrup (OTC) | Drowsiness,<br>constipation,<br>nausea, stomach<br>upset, sedation,<br>itching. | Do not take for<br>chronic cough<br>associated with<br>smoking, asthma,<br>or emphysema.<br>Care should be<br>taken when per-<br>forming tasks re-<br>quiring alertness. | | OTC Use—<br>If cough<br>continues<br>beyond 7 to 10<br>days, see a<br>doctor. |
| **Benzonatate**<br>*Tessalon Perles*<br>capsule ($R$) | May cause<br>drowsiness,<br>constipation,<br>nausea, sto-<br>mach upset,<br>sedation,<br>itching. | Do not take for<br>chronic cough<br>associated with<br>smoking,<br>asthma, or<br>emphysema. | Do not chew or<br>break capsules. | |

Respiratory

# Antiasthmatics—Miscellaneous

**ACTION** Cromolyn sodium decreases the release of chemicals into the narrow airways of the lung. Nedocromil sodium inhibits the activity of inflammatory cells associated with asthma. Ipratropium bromide antagonizes acetylcholine thus widening the air passages.

**INDICATION** Used to treat bronchial asthma.

| Generic Name<br>*Brand Name* | Side Effects | Warnings | Dosing | Notes |
|---|---|---|---|---|
| **Cromolyn Sodium**<br>*Intal* aerosol, capsules for inhalation, solution for inhalation (℞)<br>*Nasalcrom* nasal solution (OTC) | Coughing, wheezing, sneezing, nausea, nasal stinging, headache, bad taste. | Not for the treatment of an existing asthma attack. | Blow your nose before using nasal solution. Shake aerosol canister well before using. | Used for the prevention of allergic rhinitis and exercise-induced bronchospasm. Decreases severity of bronchial attacks. |
| **Nedocromil Sodium**<br>*Tilade* aerosol (℞) | Coughing, sore throat, nausea, dizziness, fatigue, diarrhea, dry mouth, stomach pain. | Not for the treatment of an existing asthma attack. | Shake aerosol canister well before using. | Used for the management of mild to moderate bronchial asthma. |
| **Ipratropium Bromide**<br>*Atrovent* aerosol, solution (℞) | Hoarseness, cough, nausea, headache, nervousness, constipation, difficult urination, blurred vision. | Not for the treatment of an existing asthma attack. Do not exceed 12 inhalations in 24 hours. | Shake aerosol canister well before using. | Used for bronchospasm occurring in chronic bronchitis, emphysema, and other obstructive disorders of the lung. |

## Antileukotriene Agents

**ACTION** Leukotrienes induce numerous biological effects that can contribute to inflammation, edema, bronchoconstriction, and mucus secretion in asthmatic patients. Zafirlukast is a leukotriene-receptor antagonist that blocks the leukotriene activity. Zileuton inhibits leukotriene formation.

**INDICATION** Prophylaxis and chronic treatment of asthma.

| Generic Name<br>*Brand Name* | Side Effects | Warnings | Dosing | Notes |
|---|---|---|---|---|
| **Zafirlukast**<br>*Accolate*<br>tablet (℞) | Headache, nausea, diarrhea, abdominal pain, dizziness, fever, vomiting. | Not for the treatment of an existing asthma attack. | Take 1 hour before or 2 hours after meals. | |
| **Zileuton**<br>*Zyflo* tablet (℞) | Headache, dyspepsia, nausea, pain, constipation, dizziness, fever. | Not for the treatment of an existing asthma attack. If fatigue, jaundice, or flu-like symptoms are experienced, contact a physician. | May take with food. Take regularly even during symptom-free periods. | |

Respiratory

# Bronchodilators—Sympathomimetics

**ACTION** Sympathomimetics relax the smooth muscle around the bronchioles (air sacs) of the lung resulting in a widening of the bronchioles. This prevents spasms or contractions of the smooth muscles, allowing for better air exchange. The release of histamine is also inhibited, which creates a positive antiallergenic effect on breathing.

**INDICATION** Used to treat reversible bronchospasm associated with asthma, bronchitis, emphysema, exercise-induced bronchospasm, and other obstructive diseases of the lung.

**BANNED SUBSTANCES** NCAA and/or USOC may list some of these substances as banned for athletes to use.

| Generic Name<br>*Brand Name* | Side Effects | Warnings | Dosing | Notes |
|---|---|---|---|---|
| **Albuterol**<br>*Proventil, Ventolin*<br>tablet, syrup (℞)<br>*Volmax, Proventil*<br>*Repetabs* extended release<br>tablet (℞)<br>*Proventil, Ventolin*<br>aerosol, solution<br>for inhalation,<br>capsules for<br>inhalation (℞) | Nervousness, restlessness, dizziness, sleeplessness, dry mouth, appetite changes. | Wait 3 to 5 minutes for second inhalation if more than one inhalation is necessary per dose. | Shake aerosol canister before using. | To prevent exercise-induced bronchospasm, use 15 minutes prior to exercise. |
| **Albuterol,**<br>**Ipratropium**<br>**Bromide**<br>*Combivent*<br>aerosol syrup<br>(℞) | Nervousness, bronchospasm, headache, bronchitis, restlessness, dizziness, sleeplessness, dry mouth, appetite changes. | Wait 3 to 5 minutes for second inhalation if more than one inhalation is necessary per dose. | Shake aerosol canister before using. | |
| **Bitolterol**<br>**Mesylate**<br>*Tornalate* aerosol,<br>solution for<br>inhalation (℞) | Nervousness, restlessness, dizziness, sleeplessness, dry mouth, appetite changes. | Wait 1 minute for second inhalation if more than one inhalation is necessary per dose. | Shake aerosol canister before using. | |

**ACTION** Sympathomimetics relax the smooth muscle around the bronchioles (air sacs) of the lung resulting in a widening of the bronchioles. This prevents spasms or contractions of the smooth muscles, allowing for better air exchange. The release of histamine is also inhibited, which creates a positive antiallergenic effect on breathing.

**INDICATION** Used to treat reversible bronchospasm associated with asthma, bronchitis, emphysema, exercise-induced bronchospasm, and other obstructive diseases of the lung.

**BANNED SUBSTANCES** NCAA and/or USOC may list some of these substances as banned for athletes to use.

| Generic Name<br>Brand Name | Side Effects | Warnings | Dosing | Notes |
|---|---|---|---|---|
| **Ephedrine Sulfate**<br>Ephedrine sulfate capsule (OTC)<br>Ephedrine sulfate capsule (℞) | Nervousness, restlessness, sleeplessness. Notify a doctor if chest pain, palpitations, flushing, or breathing difficulties occur. | | If stomach upset occurs, take with food. | OTC Use—If cough continues beyond 7 to 10 days, see a doctor. |
| **Epinephrine Sulfate**<br>Adrenalin Chloride solution for inhalation (OTC)<br>Bronkaid Mist, Primatene Mist aerosol inhaler (OTC) | Nervousness, restlessness, sleeplessness. | Wait 3 to 5 minutes for second inhalation if more than one inhalation is necessary per dose. | Shake aerosol canister before using. | |
| **Isoetharine HCl**<br>Bronkometer aerosol (℞)<br>Bronkosol solution for inhalation (℞) | Nervousness, restlessness, dizziness, sleeplessness, dry mouth, appetite changes. | Wait 1 minute for second inhalation if more than one inhalation is necessary per dose. | Shake aerosol canister before using. | |
| **Isoproterenol**<br>Isuprel, Medihaler-Iso aerosol (℞)<br>Isuprel solution for inhalation, sublingual tablets (℞) | Nervousness, restlessness, dizziness, sleeplessness, dry mouth, appetite changes. | Wait 3 to 5 minutes for second inhalation if more than one inhalation is necessary per dose. | Shake aerosol canister before using. Do not swallow tablet; let it dissolve under the tongue. | |

**ACTION** Sympathomimetics relax the smooth muscle around the bronchioles (air sacs) of the lung resulting in a widening of the bronchioles. This prevents spasms or contractions of the smooth muscles, allowing for better air exchange. The release of histamine is also inhibited, which creates a positive antiallergenic effect on breathing.

**INDICATION** Used to treat reversible bronchospasm associated with asthma, bronchitis, emphysema, exercise-induced bronchospasm, and other obstructive diseases of the lung.

**BANNED SUBSTANCES** NCAA and/or USOC may list some of these substances as banned for athletes to use.

| Generic Name<br>Brand Name | Side Effects | Warnings | Dosing | Notes |
|---|---|---|---|---|
| **Isoproterenol HCl,**<br>**Phenylephrine**<br>**Bitartrate**<br>*Duo-Medihaler*<br>aerosol (℞) | Nervousness, restlessness, dizziness, sleeplessness, dry mouth, appetite changes. | Wait 3 to 5 minutes for second inhalation if more than one inhalation is necessary per dose. | Shake aerosol canister before using. | |
| **Metaproterenol**<br>**Sulfate**<br>*Alupent, Metaprel*<br>tablet, aerosol, syrup, solution for inhalation (℞) | Nervousness, restlessness, dizziness, sleeplessness, dry mouth, appetite changes. | Wait 10 minutes for second inhalation if more than one inhalation is necessary per dose. | Shake aerosol canister before using. If tablets upset stomach, take with food. | |
| **Pirbuterol**<br>**Acetate**<br>*Maxair*<br>aerosol (℞) | Nervousness, restlessness, dizziness, sleeplessness, dry mouth, appetite changes. | Wait 1 minute for second inhalation if more than one inhalation is necessary per dose. | Shake aerosol canister before using. | |
| **Salmeterol**<br>**Xinafoate**<br>*Serevent*<br>aerosol (℞) | Nervousness, restlessness, dizziness, sleeplessness, dry mouth, appetite changes. | Wait 1 minute for second inhalation if more than one inhalation is necessary per dose. Do not exceed normal daily dosage. | Shake aerosol canister before using. | To prevent exercise-induced bronchospasm, use 30 to 60 minutes before exercise. |
| **Terbutaline**<br>**Sulfate**<br>*Brethine, Bricanyl*<br>tablet (℞)<br>*Brethine*<br>aerosol (℞) | Nervousness, restlessness, dizziness, sleeplessness, dry mouth, appetite changes. | Wait 1 minute for second inhalation if more than one inhalation is necessary per dose. | Shake aerosol canister before using. | May also be used to inhibit premature labor. |

# Bronchodilators—Xanthines

**ACTION** Xanthine derivatives relax the smooth muscle around the bronchioles (air sacs) of the lung resulting in a widening of the airway that makes breathing easier.

**INDICATION** Used to prevent, treat bronchial asthma, but is not used in an acute attack. Also used to treat bronchospasms associated with chronic bronchitis and emphysema.

Respiratory

| Generic Name<br>*Brand Name* | Side Effects | Warnings | Dosing | Notes |
|---|---|---|---|---|
| **Aminophylline**<br>*Phyllocontin*<br>controlled-release tablet (℞)<br>*Aminophylline*<br>tablet, oral liquid, rectal suppository (℞) | Headache, sleeplessness, irritability, flushing, increased urination, nausea, diarrhea, increased breathing. | Avoid large amounts of caffeine as it may increase side effects. | Take at regular intervals. May take with food if stomach upset occurs. | |
| **Dyphylline**<br>*Dilor, Lufyllin*<br>tablet, elixir (℞) | Headache, sleeplessness, irritability, flushing, increased urination, nausea, diarrhea, increased breathing. | Avoid large amounts of caffeine as it may increase side effects. | Take at regular intervals. May take with food if stomach upset occurs. | |
| **Oxtriphylline**<br>*Choledyl SA*<br>sustained-action tablet (℞)<br>*Choledyl*<br>tablet, syrup, elixir (℞) | Headache, sleeplessness, irritability, flushing, increased urination, nausea, diarrhea, increased breathing. | Avoid large amounts of caffeine as it may increase side effects. | Take at regular intervals. May take with food if stomach upset occurs. | |
| **Theophylline**<br>*Theobid, Slo-Phyllin, Theo-24, Theo-Dur, Constant-T, Quibron, Theolair* (℞) | Headache, sleeplessness, irritability, flushing, increased urination, nausea, diarrhea, increased breathing. | Avoid large amounts of caffeine as it may increase side effects. | Take at regular intervals. May take immediate-release tablets and capsules with food if stomach upset occurs. | Numerous brands are made in capsule, tablet, time-release tablet, time-release capsule, syrup, elixir, and solution. |

# Corticosteroid Inhalants

**ACTION** These steroids either prevent narrowing or relax the smooth muscle of the lung airways. They are not used to treat an acute asthma attack. When inhaled the incidence of side effects is low and the effect is localized to the lungs.

**INDICATION** Used to prevent and reduce the frequency of bronchial asthma attacks in patients requiring chronic treatment where asthma is not controlled by bronchodilators or other nonsteroid medications. Wait several minutes after using a bronchodilator before using a corticosteroid inhaler to allow better absorption into the lung airways.

**BANNED SUBSTANCES** NCAA and/or USOC may list some of these substances as banned for athletes to use.

| Generic Name<br>*Brand Name* | Side Effects | Warnings | Dosing | Notes |
|---|---|---|---|---|
| **Beclomethasone Dipropionate**<br>*Beclovent, Vanceril Double Strength* aerosol (℞) | Dry mouth, hoarseness, coughing, wheezing, fungal infections of throat, facial edema, rash. | Allow at least 1 minute between inhalations. | Shake aerosol canister well before using. Moisten throat with water before using and rinse mouth with water to reduce dry mouth and hoarseness. | Allergic reaction (e.g., rash, hives) may be immediate or delayed. |
| **Dexamethasone Sodium Phosphate**<br>*Decadron Respihaler* aerosol (℞) | Dry mouth, hoarseness, coughing, wheezing, fungal infections of throat, facial edema, rash. | Allow at least 1 minute between inhalations. | Shake aerosol canister well before using. Moisten throat with water before using and rinse mouth with water to reduce dry mouth and hoarseness. | |
| **Flunisolide**<br>*AeroBid, AeroBid-M* aerosol (℞) | Dry mouth, hoarseness, coughing, wheezing, fungal infections of throat, facial edema, rash. | Allow at least 1 minute between inhalations. | Shake aerosol canister well before using. Moisten throat with water before using and rinse mouth with water to reduce dry mouth and hoarseness. | |

**ACTION** These steroids either prevent narrowing or relax the smooth muscle of the lung airways. They are not used to treat an acute asthma attack. When inhaled the incidence of side effects is low and the effect is localized to the lungs.

**INDICATION** Used to prevent and reduce the frequency of bronchial asthma attacks in patients requiring chronic treatment where asthma is not controlled by bronchodilators or other nonsteroid medications. Wait several minutes after using a bronchodilator before using a corticosteroid inhaler to allow better absorption into the lung airways.

**BANNED SUBSTANCES** NCAA and/or USOC may list some of these substances as banned for athletes to use.

| Generic Name<br>*Brand Name* | Side Effects | Warnings | Dosing | Notes |
|---|---|---|---|---|
| **Fluticasone**<br>*Flovent*<br>aerosol ($\textrm{R}$) | Dry mouth, hoarseness, coughing, wheezing, fungal infections of throat, facial edema, rash. | Allow at least 1 to 2 minutes between inhalations. | Shake aerosol canister well before using. Moisten throat with water before using and rinse mouth with water to reduce dry mouth and hoarseness. | |
| **Triamcinolone Acetonide**<br>*Azmacort*<br>aerosol ($\textrm{R}$) | Dry mouth, hoarseness, coughing, wheezing, fungal infections of throat, facial edema, rash. | Allow at least 1 minute between inhalations. | Shake aerosol canister well before using. Moisten throat with water before using and rinse mouth with water to reduce dry mouth and hoarseness. | |

## Decongestants

**ACTION** Nasal decongestants stimulate smooth muscle of blood vessels to constrict or narrow the blood vessels and thus shrink swollen and congested mucous membranes. This relieves congestion, improves breathing, and promotes mucous drainage. Drops and sprays will cause more intense nasal vasoconstriction than tablets or liquids. Decongestants may increase blood pressure and should be used with caution in individuals with high blood pressure or other cardiovascular diseases.

**INDICATION** Used to treat nasal congestion due to allergies, common cold, hay fever, and sinusitis. Also used to treat eustachian tube congestion (plugged ears). Avoid "shotgun" therapy with combination products unless needed. Using a multiple-ingredient product when not necessary may increase the risk for side effects and drug interactions.

**BANNED SUBSTANCES** NCAA and/or USOC may list some of these substances as banned for athletes to use.

| Generic Name<br>*Brand Name* | Side Effects | Warnings | Dosing | Notes |
|---|---|---|---|---|
| **Ephedrine**<br>*Vicks Vatronol*<br>nasal drops (OTC) | Anxiety, restless-ness, sleepless-ness, nausea, appetite loss, increased blood pressure, re-bound congestion, dryness. | | | OTC—Do not use for longer than 3 to 5 days. |
| **Naphazoline**<br>*Privine* nasal<br>solution<br>(OTC) | Anxiety, restless-ness, sleepless-ness, nausea, appetite loss, increased blood pressure, re-bound conges-tion, dryness. | | | OTC—Do not use for longer than 3 to 5 days. |
| **Oxymetazoline HCl**<br>*Afrin, Dristan,*<br>*4-Way Long*<br>*Lasting,*<br>*Neo-Synephrine,*<br>*Nostrilla* nasal<br>solution (OTC) | Anxiety, restless-ness, sleepless-ness, nausea, appetite loss, increased blood pressure, re-bound conges-tion, dryness. | | | OTC—Do not use for longer than 3 to 5 days. |

**ACTION** Nasal decongestants stimulate smooth muscle of blood vessels to constrict or narrow the blood vessels and thus shrink swollen and congested mucous membranes. This relieves congestion, improves breathing, and promotes mucous drainage. Drops and sprays will cause more intense nasal vasoconstriction than tablets or liquids. Decongestants may increase blood pressure and should be used with caution in individuals with high blood pressure or other cardiovascular diseases.

**INDICATION** Used to treat nasal congestion due to allergies, common cold, hay fever, and sinusitis. Also used to treat eustachian tube congestion (plugged ears). Avoid "shotgun" therapy with combination products unless needed. Using a multiple-ingredient product when not necessary may increase the risk for side effects and drug interactions.

**BANNED SUBSTANCES** NCAA and/or USOC may list some of these substances as banned for athletes to use.

| Generic Name<br>*Brand Name* | Side Effects | Warnings | Dosing | Notes |
|---|---|---|---|---|
| **Phenylephrine HCl**<br>*AH-Chew D*<br>chewable tablet<br>(OTC)<br>*Neo-Synephrine,*<br>*Nostril, Sinex*<br>nasal solution<br>(OTC) | Anxiety, restless-ness, sleepless-ness, nausea, appetite loss, increased blood pressure, re-bound conges-tion, dryness. | | | OTC—Do not use nasal solution for longer than 3 to 5 days. |
| **Phenylpropanola-mine HCl**<br>*Propagest* tablet (OTC)<br>*Dexatrim*<br>time-release<br>capsule (OTC)<br>*Acutrim*<br>time-release<br>tablet (OTC) | Anxiety, restless-ness, sleepless-ness, nausea, appetite loss, increased blood pressure, re-bound conges-tion, dryness. | Do not exceed 150 mg in 24 hours. If symptoms do not improve in 7 days, consult a doctor. | | Phenylpropanola-mine is used in OTC appetite suppressants as an adjunct short-term treatment with calorie restrictions for weight loss. |
| **Pseudoephe-drine HCl**<br>*Sudafed* tablet (OTC)<br>*Efidac/24* extended-release tablet (OTC)<br>*Sudafed 12 Hour*<br>extended-release<br>capsule (OTC)<br>*Children's Sudafed,*<br>*Dorcol Decongestant*<br>liquid (OTC) | Anxiety, restless-ness, sleepless-ness, nausea, appetite loss, increased blood pressure, re-bound conges-tion, dryness. | Do not exceed 360 mg in 24 hours. If symptoms do not improve in 7 days, consult a doctor. | | |

**ACTION** Nasal decongestants stimulate smooth muscle of blood vessels to constrict or narrow the blood vessels and thus shrink swollen and congested mucous membranes. This relieves congestion, improves breathing, and promotes mucous drainage. Drops and sprays will cause more intense nasal vasoconstriction than tablets or liquids. Decongestants may increase blood pressure and should be used with caution in individuals with high blood pressure or other cardiovascular diseases.

**INDICATION** Used to treat nasal congestion due to allergies, common cold, hay fever, and sinusitis. Also used to treat eustachian tube congestion (plugged ears). Avoid "shotgun" therapy with combination products unless needed. Using a multiple-ingredient product when not necessary may increase the risk for side effects and drug interactions.

**BANNED SUBSTANCES** NCAA and/or USOC may list some of these substances as banned for athletes to use.

| Generic Name<br>*Brand Name* | Side Effects | Warnings | Dosing | Notes |
|---|---|---|---|---|
| **Tetrahydrozoline HCl**<br>*Tyzine* nasal solution (℞) | Anxiety, restlessness, sleeplessness, nausea, appetite loss, increased blood pressure, rebound congestion, dryness. | | | |
| **Xylometazoline HCl**<br>*Otrivin* nasal solution (OTC) | Anxiety, restlessness, sleeplessness, nausea, appetite loss, increased blood pressure, rebound congestion, dryness. | | | OTC—Do not use for longer than 3 to 5 days. |

## Expectorants

**ACTION** Expectorants increase mucous secretions and make the phlegm less sticky. The mucus then becomes easier to cough up.

**INDICATION** Used to loosen respiratory secretions and mucus. It is important to maintain a well-hydrated body by drinking plenty of fluids as this assists in thinning the mucus. Avoid "shotgun" therapy with combination products unless needed. Using a multiple-ingredient product when not necessary may increase the risk for side effects and drug interactions.

Respiratory

| Generic Name<br>Brand Name | Side Effects | Warnings | Dosing | Notes |
|---|---|---|---|---|
| **Guaifenesin**<br>*Fenesin, Humibid<br>   L.A.* sustained-<br>   release tablet (℞)<br>*Humibid Sprinkle*<br>   sustained-release<br>   capsule (℞)<br>*Robitussin, Guia-<br>   tuss, Scot-Tussin*<br>   syrup (OTC)<br>*Naldecon Senior<br>   EX* liquid (OTC) | Nausea, vomit-<br>ing, dizziness,<br>headache, rash. | Do not take for<br>chronic cough<br>associated with<br>smoking, asthma,<br>or emphysema. | Drink a full glass<br>of water or other<br>fluid with<br>each dose. | OTC Use—If<br>cough continues<br>beyond 1 week<br>see a doctor. |
| **Iodinated<br>   Glycerol**<br>*Iophen* tablet,<br>   elixir, solution<br>   (℞) | Nausea, vomit-<br>ing, dizziness,<br>headache, rash. | Do not take for<br>chronic cough<br>associated with<br>smoking, asthma,<br>or emphysema. | Drink a full glass<br>of water or other<br>fluid with<br>each dose. | |
| **Potassium Iodide**<br>*Pima, SSKI*<br>   solution, syrup<br>   (℞) | Nausea, vomit-<br>ing, dizziness,<br>headache, rash. | Do not take for<br>chronic cough<br>associated with<br>smoking, asthma,<br>or emphysema. | Drink a full glass<br>of water or other<br>fluid with<br>each dose. | |

## Intranasal Steroids

**ACTION** Intranasal steroids work by shrinking the swollen nasal tissue and reducing inflammation.

**INDICATION** Used to treat seasonal and continual allergic rhinitis or hay fever involving inflammation of the mucous membranes of the nasal passages. Allergic rhinitis symptoms include itching, runny nose, postnasal drip, sneezing, and nasal congestion. Will not significantly relieve allergic conjunctivitis (watering itchy eyes). Steroids may slow or prevent healing and should be used with caution if you have a fungal, bacterial, or viral infection.

**BANNED SUBSTANCES** NCAA and/or USOC may list some of these substances as banned for athletes to use.

| Generic Name<br>*Brand Name* | Side Effects | Warnings | Dosing | Notes |
|---|---|---|---|---|
| **Beclomethasone Dipropionate**<br>*Beconase,*<br>*Vancenase*<br>aerosol (℞)<br>*Beconase AQ,*<br>*Vancenase DS*<br>spray (℞) | Nasal and throat irritation, stinging, dryness, cough, sneezing, headache, dizziness, nausea. | Do not exceed recommended dosage. | Shake aerosol canister well before using. Blow your nose before using. | Also used for nonallergic rhinitis in adults. |
| **Budesonide**<br>*Rhinocort*<br>aerosol (℞) | Nasal and throat irritation, stinging, dryness, cough, sneezing, headache, dizziness, nausea. | Do not exceed recommended dosage. | Shake aerosol canister well before using. Blow your nose before using. | Also used for nonallergic rhinitis in adults. |
| **Dexamethasone Sodium Phosphate**<br>*Decadron*<br>*Turbinaire*<br>aerosol (℞) | Nasal and throat irritation, stinging, dryness, cough, sneezing, headache, dizziness, nausea. | Do not exceed recommended dosage. | Shake aerosol canister well before using. Blow your nose before using. | |
| **Flunisolide**<br>*Nasalide*<br>aerosol (℞) | Nasal and throat irritation, stinging, dryness, cough, sneezing, headache, dizziness, nausea. | Do not exceed recommended dosage. | Shake aerosol canister well before using. Blow your nose before using. | Also used for nonallergic rhinitis in adults. |

**ACTION** Intranasal steroids work by shrinking the swollen nasal tissue and reducing inflammation.

**INDICATION** Used to treat seasonal and continual allergic rhinitis or hay fever involving inflammation of the mucous membranes of the nasal passages. Allergic rhinitis symptoms include itching, runny nose, postnasal drip, sneezing, and nasal congestion. Will not significantly relieve allergic conjunctivitis (watering itchy eyes). Steroids may slow or prevent healing and should be used with caution if you have a fungal, bacterial, or viral infection.

**BANNED SUBSTANCES** NCAA and/or USOC may list some of these substances as banned for athletes to use.

| Generic Name<br>*Brand Name* | Side Effects | Warnings | Dosing | Notes |
|---|---|---|---|---|
| **Fluticasone Propionate**<br>*Flonase* aerosol<br>(℞) | Nasal and throat irritation, stinging, dryness, cough, sneezing, headache, dizziness, nausea. | Do not exceed recommended dosage. | Shake aerosol canister well before using. Blow your nose before using. | |
| **Triamcinolone Acetonide**<br>*Nasacort* aerosol<br>(℞)<br>*Nasacort AQ* spray<br>(℞) | Nasal and throat irritation, stinging, dryness, cough, sneezing, headache, dizziness, nausea. | Do not exceed recommended dosage. | Shake aerosol canister well before using. Blow your nose before using. | |

## Antiasthmatic Combinations

Numerous combination products are available both by prescription and over-the-counter for respiratory conditions. Often, a product may either contain ingredients not needed or the wrong strength of an ingredient that is needed. It is advisable to avoid "shotgun" therapy with combination products unless needed. Using a multiple-ingredient product when not necessary can increase the risk for side effects and drug interactions.

The following tables identify commonly used products with the ingredients contained in each. Many common brand names formerly associated with one ingredient may have several different formulations on the market. It is important to identify the ingredients in a product. Detailed information on all the ingredients included in this table is provided elsewhere in the text.

**INDICATION** These products are generally used for asthma and other breathing problems.

**BANNED SUBSTANCES** NCAA and/or USOC may list some of these substances as banned for athletes to use.

| Brand Names | Xanthine Bronchodilator | Sympathomimetic Bronchodilator | Expectorant | Other |
|---|---|---|---|---|
| Asbron (℞) | Theophylline | | Guaifenesin | |
| Bronkaid (OTC) | Theophylline | Ephedrine | Guaifenesin | |
| Bronkolixir (OTC) | Theophylline | Ephedrine | Guaifenesin | Phenobarbital |
| Bronkotabs (OTC) | Theophylline | Ephedrine | Guaifenesin | Phenobarbital |
| Dilor-G Elixir (℞) | Dyphylline | | Guaifenesin | |
| Dilor-G (℞) | Theophylline | | Guaifenesin | |
| Elixophyllin-Potassium Iodide (℞) | Theophylline | | Potassium Iodide | |
| Hydrophed (℞) | Theophylline | Ephedrine | | Hydroxyzine HCl |
| Iophylline (℞) | Theophylline | | Guaifenesin | |
| Lufyllin-GG Elixir (℞) | Dyphylline | | Guaifenesin | |
| Lufyllin-GG (℞) | Theophylline | | Guaifenesin | |
| Marax (℞) | Theophylline | Ephedrine | | Hydroxyzine HCl |
| Marax-DF (℞) | Theophylline | Ephedrine | | Hydroxyzine HCl |
| Mudrane GG (℞) | Theophylline | Ephedrine | Guaifenesin | Phenobarbital |
| Mudrane (℞) | Theophylline | Ephedrine | Potassium Iodide | Phenobarbital |

Numerous combination products are available both by prescription and over-the-counter for respiratory conditions. Often, a product may either contain ingredients not needed or the wrong strength of an ingredient that is needed. It is advisable to avoid "shotgun" therapy with combination products unless needed. Using a multiple-ingredient product when not necessary can increase the risk for side effects and drug interactions.

The following tables identify commonly used products with the ingredients contained in each. Many common brand names formerly associated with one ingredient may have several different formulations on the market. It is important to identify the ingredients in a product. Detailed information on all the ingredients included in this table is provided elsewhere in the text.

**INDICATION** These products are generally used for asthma and other breathing problems.

**BANNED SUBSTANCES** NCAA and/or USOC may list some of these substances as banned for athletes to use.

| Brand Names | Xanthine Bronchodilator | Sympathomimetic Bronchodilator | Expectorant | Other |
|---|---|---|---|---|
| Primatene (OTC) | Theophylline | Ephedrine | | |
| Primatene Dual Action (OTC) | Theophylline | Ephedrine | Guaifenesin | |
| Quadrinal (Rx) | Theophylline | Ephedrine | Potassium Iodide | Phenobarbital |
| Quibron (Rx) | Theophylline | | Guaifenesin | |
| Slo-Phyllin GG (Rx) | Theophylline | | Guaifenesin | |
| Theomax DF (Rx) | Theophylline | Ephedrine | | Hydroxyzine HCl |
| Theophylline-Organidin (Rx) | Theophylline | | Guaifenesin | |

Respiratory

## Cough Combinations

Numerous combination products are available both by prescription and over-the-counter for respiratory conditions. Often a product may either contain ingredients not needed or the wrong strength of an ingredient that is needed. It is advisable to avoid "shotgun" therapy with combination products unless needed. Using a multiple-ingredient product when not necessary can increase the risk for side effects and drug interactions.

The following tables identify commonly used products with the ingredients contained in each. Many common brand names formerly associated with one ingredient may have several different formulations on the market. It is important to identify the ingredients in a product. Detailed information on all the ingredients included in this table is provided elsewhere in the text.

**INDICATION** These products are generally used for cough and cold symptoms.

**BANNED SUBSTANCES** NCAA and/or USOC may list some of these substances as banned for athletes to use. Decongestants and caffeine may be based on urine concentrations and use.

| Brand Names | Antitussive | Decongestant | Antihistamine | Other |
|---|---|---|---|---|
| Actagen-C (℞, C-V) | Codeine Phosphate | Pseudoephedrine HCl | Triprolidine HCl | |
| Actifed w/Codeine (℞, C-V) | Codeine Phosphate | Pseudoephedrine HCl | Triprolidine HCl | |
| Alka-Seltzer Plus Cold & Cough (OTC) | Dextromethorphan HBr | Phenylpropanolamine HCl Bitartrate | Chlorpheniramine Maleate | Aspirin, Phenylalanine |
| Alka-Seltzer Plus Night-Time Cold (OTC) | Dextromethorphan HBr | Pseudoephedrine HCl | Doxylamine Succinate | Acetaminophen |
| Ambenyl Cough (C-V) | Codeine Phosphate | | Bromodiphenhydramine HCl | |
| Ambenyl-D (OTC) | Dextromethorphan HBr | Pseudoephedrine HCl | | Guaifenesin |
| Anaplex HD (℞, C-III) | Hydrocodone Bitartrate | Phenylephrine HCl | Chlorpheniramine Maleate | |
| Anatuss (OTC) | Dextromethorphan HBr | Phenylpropanolamine HCl | | Guaifenesin |
| Anatuss LA (℞) | | Pseudoephedrine HCl | | Guaifenesin |
| Bayer Select Night Time Cold (OTC) | Dextromethorphan HBr | Pseudoephedrine HCl | Triprolidine HCl | Acetaminophen |

Numerous combination products are available both by prescription and over-the-counter for respiratory conditions. Often a product may either contain ingredients not needed or the wrong strength of an ingredient that is needed. It is advisable to avoid "shotgun" therapy with combination products unless needed. Using a multiple-ingredient product when not necessary can increase the risk for side effects and drug interactions.

The following tables identify commonly used products with the ingredients contained in each. Many common brand names formerly associated with one ingredient may have several different formulations on the market. It is important to identify the ingredients in a product. Detailed information on all the ingredients included in this table is provided elsewhere in the text.

**INDICATION** These products are generally used for cough and cold symptoms.

**BANNED SUBSTANCES** NCAA and/or USOC may list some of these substances as banned for athletes to use. Decongestants and caffeine may be based on urine concentrations and use.

| Brand Names | Antitussive | Decongestant | Antihistamine | Other |
|---|---|---|---|---|
| Benylin Expectorant (OTC) | Dextrometh-orphan HBr | | | Guaifenesin |
| Bromotuss w/ Codeine (℞, C-V) | Codeine Phosphate | | Bromodiphen-hydramine HCl | |
| Bromphen DX (℞) | Dextrometh-orphan HBr | Pseudoephed-rine HCl | Brompheni ra-mine Maleate | |
| Bromphen DC w/ Codeine (℞, C-V) | Codeine Phosphate | Phenylpropa-nolamine HCl | Brompheni ra-mine Maleate | |
| Bronkaid Dual Action (OTC) | | Ephedrine | | Guaifenesin |
| Bronkolate (℞) | | Ephedrine | | Guaifenesin |
| Brontex (℞, C-V) | Codeine Phosphate | | | Guaifenesin |
| Calcidrine (℞, C-V) | Codeine Phosphate | | | Calcium Iodide |
| Carbodec DM (℞) | Dextrometh-orphan HBr | Pseudoephed-rine HCl | Carbinoxa-mine Maleate | |
| Cardec DM (℞) | Dextrometh-orphan HBr | Pseudoephed-rine HCl | Carbinoxa-mine Maleate | |
| Cerose-DM (OTC) | Dextrometh-orphan HBr | Phenylpropa-nolamine HCl | Carbinoxa-mine Maleate | |
| Cheracol Plus 1 (OTC) | Dextrometh-orphan HBr | Phenylpropa-nolamine HCl | Chlorpheni ra-mine Maleate | |

Numerous combination products are available both by prescription and over-the-counter for respiratory conditions. Often a product may either contain ingredients not needed or the wrong strength of an ingredient that is needed. It is advisable to avoid "shotgun" therapy with combination products unless needed. Using a multiple-ingredient product when not necessary can increase the risk for side effects and drug interactions.

The following tables identify commonly used products with the ingredients contained in each. Many common brand names formerly associated with one ingredient may have several different formulations on the market. It is important to identify the ingredients in a product. Detailed information on all the ingredients included in this table is provided elsewhere in the text.

**INDICATION** These products are generally used for cough and cold symptoms.

**BANNED SUBSTANCES** NCAA and/or USOC may list some of these substances as banned for athletes to use. Decongestants and caffeine may be based on urine concentrations and use.

| Brand Names | Antitussive | Decongestant | Antihistamine | Other |
|---|---|---|---|---|
| Cheracol Cough (℞, C-V) | Codeine Phosphate | | | Guaifenesin |
| Cheracol-D (OTC) | Dextromethorphan HBr | | | Guaifenesin |
| Codamine (℞, C-III) | Hydrocodone Bitartrate | Phenylpropanolamine HCl | | |
| Codehist DH (℞, C-V) | Codeine Phosphate | Pseudoephedrine HCl | Chlorpheniramine Maleate | |
| Codiclear DH (℞, C-III) | Hydrocodone Bitartrate | | | Guaifenesin |
| Codimal PH (℞, C-V) | Codeine Phosphate | Phenylephrine HCl | Pyrilamine Maleate | |
| Codimal DH (℞, C-III) | Hydrocodone Bitartrate | Phenylephrine HCl | Pyrilamine Maleate | |
| Codimal DM (OTC) | Dextromethorphan HBr | Phenylephrine HCl | Pyrilamine Maleate | |
| Comtrex Liqui-Gels (OTC) | Dextromethorphan HBr | Phenylpropanolamine HCl | Chlorpheniramine Maleate | Acetaminophen |
| Comtrex (OTC) | Dextromethorphan HBr | Pseudoephedrine HCl | Chlorpheniramine Maleate | Acetaminophen |
| Congestac (OTC) | | Pseudoephedrine HCl | | Guaifenesin |

Numerous combination products are available both by prescription and over-the-counter for respiratory conditions. Often a product may either contain ingredients not needed or the wrong strength of an ingredient that is needed. It is advisable to avoid "shotgun" therapy with combination products unless needed. Using a multiple-ingredient product when not necessary can increase the risk for side effects and drug interactions.

The following tables identify commonly used products with the ingredients contained in each. Many common brand names formerly associated with one ingredient may have several different formulations on the market. It is important to identify the ingredients in a product. Detailed information on all the ingredients included in this table is provided elsewhere in the text.

**INDICATION** These products are generally used for cough and cold symptoms.

**BANNED SUBSTANCES** NCAA and/or USOC may list some of these substances as banned for athletes to use. Decongestants and caffeine may be based on urine concentrations and use.

| Brand Names | Antitussive | Decongestant | Antihistamine | Other |
|---|---|---|---|---|
| Contac Severe Cold & Flu (OTC) | Dextromethorphan HBr | Pseudoephedrine HCl | Chlorpheniramine Maleate | Acetaminophen |
| Contact Severe Cold & Flu Formula (OTC) | Dextromethorphan HBr | Phenylpropanolamine HCl | Chlorpheniramine Maleate | Acetaminophen |
| Contact Night Cold & Flu (OTC) | Dextromethorphan HBr | Pseudoephedrine HCl | Diphenhydramine HCl | Acetaminophen |
| Deconsal II (℞) | | Pseudoephedrine HCl | | Guaifenesin |
| Deconsal Sprinkle (℞) | | Phenylephrine HCl | | Guaifenesin |
| Dimetane DX (℞) | Dextromethorphan HBr | Pseudoephedrine HCl | Brompheniramine Maleate | |
| Dimetane DC (℞, C-V) | Codeine Phosphate | Phenylpropanolamine HCl | Brompheniramine Maleate | |
| Dimetapp DM (OTC) | Dextromethorphan HBr | Phenylpropanolamine HCl | Brompheniramine Maleate | |
| Drixoral Cough & Cold (OTC) | Dextromethorphan HBr | | | Acetaminophen |
| Dura-Vent (℞) | | Phenylpropanolamine HCl | | Guaifenesin |
| Duratuss (℞) | | Pseudoephedrine HCl | | Guaifenesin |

Numerous combination products are available both by prescription and over-the-counter for respiratory conditions. Often a product may either contain ingredients not needed or the wrong strength of an ingredient that is needed. It is advisable to avoid "shotgun" therapy with combination products unless needed. Using a multiple-ingredient product when not necessary can increase the risk for side effects and drug interactions.

The following tables identify commonly used products with the ingredients contained in each. Many common brand names formerly associated with one ingredient may have several different formulations on the market. It is important to identify the ingredients in a product. Detailed information on all the ingredients included in this table is provided elsewhere in the text.

**INDICATION** These products are generally used for cough and cold symptoms.

**BANNED SUBSTANCES** NCAA and/or USOC may list some of these substances as banned for athletes to use. Decongestants and caffeine may be based on urine concentrations and use.

| Brand Names | Antitussive | Decongestant | Antihistamine | Other |
|---|---|---|---|---|
| Duratuss HD (℞, C-III) | Hydrocodone Bitartrate | Pseudoephed-rine HCl | | Guaifenesin |
| Endal Expectorant (℞, C-V) | Codeine Phosphate | Phenylpropa-nolamine HCl | | Guaifenesin |
| Endal (℞) | | Phenylephrine HCl | | Guaifenesin |
| Endal-HD Plus (℞, C-III) | Hydrocodone Bitartrate | Phenylephrine HCl | Chlorphenira-mine Maleate | |
| Endal-HD (℞, C-III) | Hydrocodone Bitartrate | Phenylephrine HCl | Chlorphenira-mine Maleate | |
| Entex LA (℞) | | Phenylpropa-nolamine HCl | | Guaifenesin |
| Entex PSE (℞) | | Pseudoephed-rine HCl | | Guaifenesin |
| Entex (℞) | | Phenylpropa-nolamine HCl, Phenylephrine HCl | | Guaifenesin |
| Entuss Expectorant (℞, C-III) | Hydrocodone Bitartrate | | | Potassium Guaiacol-sulfonate |
| Entuss-D (℞, C-III) | Hydrocodone Bitartrate | Pseudoephed-rine HCl | | Guaifenesin |

Numerous combination products are available both by prescription and over-the-counter for respiratory conditions. Often a product may either contain ingredients not needed or the wrong strength of an ingredient that is needed. It is advisable to avoid "shotgun" therapy with combination products unless needed. Using a multiple-ingredient product when not necessary can increase the risk for side effects and drug interactions.

The following tables identify commonly used products with the ingredients contained in each. Many common brand names formerly associated with one ingredient may have several different formulations on the market. It is important to identify the ingredients in a product. Detailed information on all the ingredients included in this table is provided elsewhere in the text.

**INDICATION** These products are generally used for cough and cold symptoms.

**BANNED SUBSTANCES** NCAA and/or USOC may list some of these substances as banned for athletes to use. Decongestants and caffeine may be based on urine concentrations and use.

| Brand Names | Antitussive | Decongestant | Antihistamine | Other |
|---|---|---|---|---|
| Fenesin DM (℞) | Dextromethorphan HBr | | | Guaifenesin |
| Guaimax-D (℞) | | Pseudoephedrine HCl | | Guaifenesin |
| Guaitab (OTC) | | Pseudoephedrine HCl | | Guaifenesin |
| Guiatuss DAC (℞, C-V) | Codeine Phosphate | Pseudoephedrine HCl | | Guaifenesin |
| Guiatuss AC (℞, C-V) | Codeine Phosphate | | | Guaifenesin |
| Histine DM (℞) | Dextromethorphan HBr | Phenylpropanolamine HCl | Brompheniramine Maleate | |
| Histinex PV (℞, C-III) | Hydrocodone Bitartrate | Pseudoephedrine HCl | Chlorpheniramine Maleate | |
| Histussin HC (℞, C-III) | Hydrocodone Bitartrate | Phenylephrine HCl | Chlorpheniramine Maleate | |
| Humibid DM (℞) | Dextromethorphan HBr | | | Guaifenesin |
| Hycodan (℞, C-III) | Hydrocodone Bitartrate | | | Homatropine MBR |
| Hycomine (℞, C-III) | Hydrocodone Bitartrate | Phenylpropanolamine HCl | | |
| Hycomine Compound (℞, C-III) | Hydrocodone Bitartrate | Phenylephrine HCl | Chlorpheniramine Maleate | Acetaminophen, Caffeine |

Respiratory

Numerous combination products are available both by prescription and over-the-counter for respiratory conditions. Often a product may either contain ingredients not needed or the wrong strength of an ingredient that is needed. It is advisable to avoid "shotgun" therapy with combination products unless needed. Using a multiple-ingredient product when not necessary can increase the risk for side effects and drug interactions.

The following tables identify commonly used products with the ingredients contained in each. Many common brand names formerly associated with one ingredient may have several different formulations on the market. It is important to identify the ingredients in a product. Detailed information on all the ingredients included in this table is provided elsewhere in the text.

**INDICATION** These products are generally used for cough and cold symptoms.

**BANNED SUBSTANCES** NCAA and/or USOC may list some of these substances as banned for athletes to use. Decongestants and caffeine may be based on urine concentrations and use.

| Brand Names | Antitussive | Decongestant | Antihistamine | Other |
|---|---|---|---|---|
| Hydromet (℞, C-III) | Hydrocodone Bitartrate | | | Homatropine MBR |
| Iophen-C (℞, C-V) | Codeine Phosphate | | | Iodinated Glycerol |
| Iophen-DM (℞) | Dextromethorphan HBr | | | Iodinated Glycerol |
| Medi-Flu (OTC) | Dextromethorphan HBr | Pseudoephedrine HCl | Chlorpheniramine Maleate | Acetaminophen |
| Multi-Symptom Tylenol Cold (OTC) | Dextromethorphan HBr | Pseudoephedrine HCl | Chlorpheniramine Maleate | Acetaminophen |
| Myphetane DX (℞) | Dextromethorphan HBr | Pseudoephedrine HCl | Brompheniramine Maleate | |
| Myphetane DC (℞, C-V) | Codeine Phosphate | Phenylpropanolamine HCl | Brompheniramine Maleate | |
| Naldecon Senior (OTC) | Dextromethorphan HBr | | | Guaifenesin |
| Naldecon CX (℞, C-V) | Codeine Phosphate | Phenylpropanolamine HCl | | Guaifenesin |
| Nasabid (℞) | | Pseudoephedrine HCl | | Guaifenesin |
| Novahistine Expectorant (℞, C-V) | Codeine Phosphate | Pseudoephedrine HCl | | Guaifenesin |
| Novahistine DH (℞, C-V) | Codeine Phosphate | Pseudoephedrine HCl | Chlorpheniramine Maleate | |

Numerous combination products are available both by prescription and over-the-counter for respiratory conditions. Often a product may either contain ingredients not needed or the wrong strength of an ingredient that is needed. It is advisable to avoid "shotgun" therapy with combination products unless needed. Using a multiple-ingredient product when not necessary can increase the risk for side effects and drug interactions.

The following tables identify commonly used products with the ingredients contained in each. Many common brand names formerly associated with one ingredient may have several different formulations on the market. It is important to identify the ingredients in a product. Detailed information on all the ingredients included in this table is provided elsewhere in the text.

**INDICATION** These products are generally used for cough and cold symptoms.

**BANNED SUBSTANCES** NCAA and/or USOC may list some of these substances as banned for athletes to use. Decongestants and caffeine may be based on urine concentrations and use.

| Brand Names | Antitussive | Decongestant | Antihistamine | Other |
|---|---|---|---|---|
| Novahistine DMX (OTC) | Dextromethorphan HBr | Pseudoephedrine HCl | | Guaifenesin |
| Nucofed (℞, C-III) | Codeine Phosphate | Pseudoephedrine HCl | | |
| Nucofed Expectorant (℞, C-V) | Codeine Phosphate | Pseudoephedrine HCl | | Guaifenesin |
| NyQuil Hot Therapy (OTC) | Dextromethorphan HBr | Pseudoephedrine HCl | Doxylamine Succinate | Acetaminophen |
| NyQuil Nighttime Cold/Flu (OTC) | Dextromethorphan HBr | Pseudoephedrine HCl | Doxylamine Succinate | |
| Ordrine AT (℞) | Caramiphen Edisylate | Phenylpropanolamine HCl | | |
| Ornex Severe Cold (OTC) | Dextromethorphan HBr | Pseudoephedrine HCl | | Acetaminophen |
| P-V-Tussin (℞, C-III) | Hydrocodone Bitartrate | Phenindamine Tartrate | | Guaifenesin |
| P-V-Tussin (℞, C-III) | Hydrocodone Bitartrate | Pseudoephedrine HCl | Chlorpheniramine Maleate | |
| Phenergan w/ Codeine (℞, C-V) | Codeine Phosphate | | Promethazine HCl | |
| Phenergan DM (℞) | Dextromethorphan HBr | | Promethazine HCl | |
| Phenergan VC w/ Codeine (℞, C-V) | Codeine Phosphate | Phenylephrine HCl | Promethazine HCl | |

Numerous combination products are available both by prescription and over-the-counter for respiratory conditions. Often a product may either contain ingredients not needed or the wrong strength of an ingredient that is needed. It is advisable to avoid "shotgun" therapy with combination products unless needed. Using a multiple-ingredient product when not necessary can increase the risk for side effects and drug interactions.

The following tables identify commonly used products with the ingredients contained in each. Many common brand names formerly associated with one ingredient may have several different formulations on the market. It is important to identify the ingredients in a product. Detailed information on all the ingredients included in this table is provided elsewhere in the text.

**INDICATION** These products are generally used for cough and cold symptoms.

**BANNED SUBSTANCES** NCAA and/or USOC may list some of these substances as banned for athletes to use. Decongestants and caffeine may be based on urine concentrations and use.

| Brand Names | Antitussive | Decongestant | Antihistamine | Other |
|---|---|---|---|---|
| Polaramine Expectorant (℞) | | Pseudoephed-rine Sulfate | Dexchlorpheni-ramine Maleate | Guaifenesin |
| Poly-Histine CS (℞, C-V) | Codeine Phosphate | Phenylpropa-nolamine HCl | Bromphenira-mine Maleate | |
| Poly-Histine DM (℞) | Dextrometh-orphan HBr | Phenylpropa-nolamine HCl | Bromphenira-mine Maleate | |
| Prometh w/Codeine (℞, C-V) | Codeine Phosphate | | Promethazine HCl | |
| Prometh VC w/ Codeine (℞, C-V) | Codeine Phosphate | Phenylephrine HCl | Promethazine HCl | |
| Prometh DM (℞) | Dextrometh-orphan HBr | | Promethazine HCl | |
| Protuss (℞, C-III) | Hydrocodone Bitartrate | | | Potassium Guaiacol-sulfonate |
| Remcol-C (OTC) | Dextrometh-orphan HBr | | Chlorphenira-mine Maleate | Acetaminophen |
| Rescaps-D (℞) | Caramiphen Edisylate | Phenylpropa-nolamine HCl | | |
| Rescon-DM (OTC) | Dextrometh-orphan HBr | Pseudoephed-rine HCl | Chlorphenira-mine Maleate | |
| Rhinosyn-DM (OTC) | Dextrometh-orphan HBr | Pseudoephed-rine HCl | Chlorphenira-mine Maleate | |

Numerous combination products are available both by prescription and over-the-counter for respiratory conditions. Often a product may either contain ingredients not needed or the wrong strength of an ingredient that is needed. It is advisable to avoid "shotgun" therapy with combination products unless needed. Using a multiple-ingredient product when not necessary can increase the risk for side effects and drug interactions.

The following tables identify commonly used products with the ingredients contained in each. Many common brand names formerly associated with one ingredient may have several different formulations on the market. It is important to identify the ingredients in a product. Detailed information on all the ingredients included in this table is provided elsewhere in the text.

**INDICATION** These products are generally used for cough and cold symptoms.

**BANNED SUBSTANCES** NCAA and/or USOC may list some of these substances as banned for athletes to use. Decongestants and caffeine may be based on urine concentrations and use.

| Brand Names | Antitussive | Decongestant | Antihistamine | Other |
|---|---|---|---|---|
| Robitussin DAC (℞, C-V) | Codeine Phosphate | Pseudoephedrine HCl | | Guaifenesin |
| Robitussin AC (℞, C-V) | Codeine Phosphate | | | Guaifenesin |
| Robitussin DM (OTC) | Dextromethorphan HBr | | | Guaifenesin |
| Robitussin PE (OTC) | | Pseudoephedrine HCl | | Guaifenesin |
| Robitussin Night Relief (OTC) | Dextromethorphan HBr | Pseudoephedrine HCl | Pyrilamine Maleate | |
| Robitussin Cough & Cold (OTC) | Dextromethorphan HBr | Pseudoephedrine HCl | | |
| Robitussin-CF (OTC) | Dextromethorphan HBr | Phenylpropanolamine HCl | | Guaifenesin |
| Rondec-DM (℞) | Dextromethorphan HBr | Pseudoephedrine HCl | Carbinoxamine Maleate | |
| Ru-Tuss with Hydrocodone (℞, C-III) | Hydrocodone Bitartrate | Phenylpropanolamine HCl, Phenylephrine HCl | Pyrilamine Maleate, Pheniramine Maleate | |
| Ru-Tuss Expectorant (OTC) | Dextromethorphan HBr | Pseudoephedrine HCl | | Guaifenesin |
| Rutuss DE (℞) | | Pseudoephedrine HCl | | Guaifenesin |

Numerous combination products are available both by prescription and over-the-counter for respiratory conditions. Often a product may either contain ingredients not needed or the wrong strength of an ingredient that is needed. It is advisable to avoid "shotgun" therapy with combination products unless needed. Using a multiple-ingredient product when not necessary can increase the risk for side effects and drug interactions.

The following tables identify commonly used products with the ingredients contained in each. Many common brand names formerly associated with one ingredient may have several different formulations on the market. It is important to identify the ingredients in a product. Detailed information on all the ingredients included in this table is provided elsewhere in the text.

**INDICATION** These products are generally used for cough and cold symptoms.

**BANNED SUBSTANCES** NCAA and/or USOC may list some of these substances as banned for athletes to use. Decongestants and caffeine may be based on urine concentrations and use.

| Brand Names | Antitussive | Decongestant | Antihistamine | Other |
|---|---|---|---|---|
| Ryna-C (℞, C-V) | Codeine Phosphate | Pseudoephedrine HCl | Chlorpheniramine Maleate | |
| Rynatuss (℞) | Carbetapentane Tannate | Phenylephrine Tannate, Ephedrine Tannate | Chlorpheniramine Tannate | |
| Scot-Tussin DM (OTC) | Dextromethorphan HBr | | Chlorpheniramine Maleate | |
| SINUvent (℞) | | Phenylpropanolamine HCl | | Guaifenesin |
| Sudafed Cough (OTC) | Dextromethorphan HBr | Pseudoephedrine HCl | | Guaifenesin |
| Sudafed Severe Cold (OTC) | Dextromethorphan HBr | Pseudoephedrine HCl | | Acetaminophen |
| Thera-Flu Non-Drowsy (OTC) | Dextromethorphan HBr | Pseudoephedrine HCl | | Acetaminophen |
| Triafed w/Codeine (℞, C-V) | Codeine Phosphate | Pseudoephedrine HCl | Triprolidine HCl | |
| Triaminic Expectorant (OTC) | | Phenylpropanolamine HCl | | Guaifenesin |
| Triaminic-DM (OTC) | Dextromethorphan HBr | Phenylpropanolamine HCl | | |
| Triaminicol Multi-Symptom Cold (OTC) | Dextromethorphan HBr | Phenylpropanolamine HCl | Chlorpheniramine Maleate | |

Numerous combination products are available both by prescription and over-the-counter for respiratory conditions. Often a product may either contain ingredients not needed or the wrong strength of an ingredient that is needed. It is advisable to avoid "shotgun" therapy with combination products unless needed. Using a multiple-ingredient product when not necessary can increase the risk for side effects and drug interactions.

The following tables identify commonly used products with the ingredients contained in each. Many common brand names formerly associated with one ingredient may have several different formulations on the market. It is important to identify the ingredients in a product. Detailed information on all the ingredients included in this table is provided elsewhere in the text.

**INDICATION** These products are generally used for cough and cold symptoms.

**BANNED SUBSTANCES** NCAA and/or USOC may list some of these substances as banned for athletes to use. Decongestants and caffeine may be based on urine concentrations and use.

| Brand Names | Antitussive | Decongestant | Antihistamine | Other |
|---|---|---|---|---|
| *Tricodene Cough & Cold* (R, C-V) | **Codeine Phosphate** | | **Pyrilamine Maleate** | |
| *Tricodene SF* (OTC) | **Dextromethorphan HBr** | | **Chlorpheniramine Maleate** | |
| *Tusquelin* (R) | **Dextromethorphan HBr** | **Phenylpropanolamine HCl, Phenylephrine HCl** | **Chlorpheniramine Maleate** | |
| *Tuss-Ornade* (R) | **Caramiphen Edisylate** | **Phenylpropanolamine HCl** | | |
| *Tussgen* (R, C-III) | **Hydrocodone Bitartrate** | **Pseudoephedrine HCl** | | |
| *Tussi-Organidin DM NR* (R) | **Dextromethorphan HBr** | | | **Guaifenesin** |
| *Tussi-Organidin NR* (R, C-V) | **Codeine Phosphate** | | | **Guaifenesin** |
| *Tussigon* (R, C-III) | **Hydrocodone Bitartrate** | | | **Homatropine MBR** |
| *Tussionex Pennkinetic* (R, C-III) | **Hydrocodone Polistirex** | | **Chlorpheniramine Maleate** | |
| *Tusso-DM* (R) | **Dextromethorphan HBr** | | | **Iodinated Glycerol** |
| *Ty-Cold* (OTC) | **Dextromethorphan HBr** | **Pseudoephedrine HCl** | **Chlorpheniramine Maleate** | **Acetaminophen** |

Respiratory

Numerous combination products are available both by prescription and over-the-counter for respiratory conditions. Often a product may either contain ingredients not needed or the wrong strength of an ingredient that is needed. It is advisable to avoid "shotgun" therapy with combination products unless needed. Using a multiple-ingredient product when not necessary can increase the risk for side effects and drug interactions.

The following tables identify commonly used products with the ingredients contained in each. Many common brand names formerly associated with one ingredient may have several different formulations on the market. It is important to identify the ingredients in a product. Detailed information on all the ingredients included in this table is provided elsewhere in the text.

**INDICATION** These products are generally used for cough and cold symptoms.

**BANNED SUBSTANCES** NCAA and/or USOC may list some of these substances as banned for athletes to use. Decongestants and caffeine may be based on urine concentrations and use.

| Brand Names | Antitussive | Decongestant | Antihistamine | Other |
|---|---|---|---|---|
| Tylenol Flu (OTC) | Dextromethorphan HBr | Pseudoephedrine HCl | | Acetaminophen |
| Vanex Expectorant (℞, C-III) | Hydrocodone Bitartrate | Pseudoephedrine HCl | | Guaifenesin |
| Vanex-HD (℞, C-III) | Hydrocodone Bitartrate | Phenylephrine HCl | Chlorpheniramine Maleate | |
| Vanex-LA (℞) | | Phenylpropanolamine HCl | | Guaifenesin |
| Vicks 44D Cough & Decongestant (OTC) | Dextromethorphan HBr | Pseudoephedrine HCl | | |
| Vicodin Tuss (℞, C-III) | Hydrocodone Bitartrate | | | Guaifenesin |
| Viro-Med (OTC) | Dextromethorphan HBr | Pseudoephedrine HCl | Chlorpheniramine Maleate | Acetaminophen |
| Zephrex (℞) | | Pseudoephedrine HCl | | Guaifenesin |

# Upper Respiratory Combinations

Numerous combination products are available both by prescription and over-the-counter for respiratory conditions. Often a product may either contain ingredients not needed or the wrong strength of an ingredient that is needed. It is advisable to avoid "shotgun" therapy with combination products unless needed. Using a multiple-ingredient product when not necessary can increase the risk for side effects and drug interactions.

The following tables identify commonly used products with the ingredients contained in each. Many common brand names formerly associated with one ingredient may have several different formulations on the market. It is important to identify the ingredients in a product. Detailed information on all the ingredients included in this table is provided elsewhere in the text.

**INDICATION** These products are generally used for runny noses, head congestion, sinus headaches, and sneezing.

**BANNED SUBSTANCES** NCAA and/or USOC may list some of these substances as banned for athletes to use.

| Brand Name | Antihistamine | Decongestant | Analgesic/Other |
|---|---|---|---|
| A.R.M. (OTC) | Chlorpheniramine Maleate | Phenylpropanolamine HCl | |
| Aceta-Gesic (OTC) | Phenyltoloxamine Citrate | | Acetaminophen |
| Actagen (OTC) | Triprolidine HCl | Pseudoephedrine HCl | |
| Actifed Plus (OTC) | Triprolidine HCl | Pseudoephedrine HCl | Acetaminophen |
| Actifed Sinus Nighttime (OTC) | Diphenhydramine HCl | Pseudoephedrine HCl | Acetaminophen |
| Actifed Allergy Nighttime (OTC) | Diphenhydramine HCl | Pseudoephedrine HCl | |
| Actifed (OTC) | Triprolidine HCl | Pseudoephedrine HCl | |
| Advil Cold & Sinus (OTC) | | Pseudoephedrine HCl | Ibuprofen |
| Alka-Seltzer Plus Cold (OTC) | Chlorpheniramine Maleate | Phenylpropanolamine HCl | Aspirin |
| Alka-Seltzer Plus Sinus (OTC) | Brompheniramine Maleate | Phenylpropanolamine HCl | Aspirin |
| Allerest (OTC) | Chlorpheniramine Maleate | Phenylpropanolamine HCl | |

Respiratory

Numerous combination products are available both by prescription and over-the-counter for respiratory conditions. Often a product may either contain ingredients not needed or the wrong strength of an ingredient that is needed. It is advisable to avoid "shotgun" therapy with combination products unless needed. Using a multiple-ingredient product when not necessary can increase the risk for side effects and drug interactions.

The following tables identify commonly used products with the ingredients contained in each. Many common brand names formerly associated with one ingredient may have several different formulations on the market. It is important to identify the ingredients in a product. Detailed information on all the ingredients included in this table is provided elsewhere in the text.

**INDICATION** These products are generally used for runny noses, head congestion, sinus headaches, and sneezing.

**BANNED SUBSTANCES** NCAA and/or USOC may list some of these substances as banned for athletes to use.

| Brand Name | Antihistamine | Decongestant | Analgesic/Other |
|---|---|---|---|
| Anamine (R) | Chlorpheniramine Maleate | Pseudoephedrine HCl | |
| Atrohist Plus (R) | Chlorpheniramine Maleate | Phenylpropanolamine HCl, Phenylephrine HCl | Belladonna Alkaloids |
| BC Cold-Sinus Powder (OTC) | | Phenylpropanolamine HCl | Aspirin |
| BC Multi Symptom Cold Powder (OTC) | Chlorpheniramine Maleate | Phenylpropanolamine HCl | Aspirin |
| Benadryl Decongestant (OTC) | Diphenhydramine HCl | Pseudoephedrine HCl | |
| Benadryl Cold (OTC) | Diphenhydramine HCl | Pseudoephedrine HCl | Acetaminophen |
| Benylin Decongestant Liquid (OTC) | Diphenhydramine HCl | Pseudoephedrine HCl | |
| Brexin LA (R) | Chlorpheniramine Maleate | Pseudoephedrine HCl | |
| Bromatapp (OTC) | Brompheniramine Maleate | Phenylpropanolamine HCl | |
| Bromfed (R) | Brompheniramine Maleate | Pseudoephedrine HCl | |
| Bromfed-PD (R) | Brompheniramine Maleate | Pseudoephedrine HCl | |

Numerous combination products are available both by prescription and over-the-counter for respiratory conditions. Often a product may either contain ingredients not needed or the wrong strength of an ingredient that is needed. It is advisable to avoid "shotgun" therapy with combination products unless needed. Using a multiple-ingredient product when not necessary can increase the risk for side effects and drug interactions.

The following tables identify commonly used products with the ingredients contained in each. Many common brand names formerly associated with one ingredient may have several different formulations on the market. It is important to identify the ingredients in a product. Detailed information on all the ingredients included in this table is provided elsewhere in the text.

**INDICATION** These products are generally used for runny noses, head congestion, sinus headaches, and sneezing.

**BANNED SUBSTANCES** NCAA and/or USOC may list some of these substances as banned for athletes to use.

| Brand Name | Antihistamine | Decongestant | Analgesic/Other |
|---|---|---|---|
| Bromphen (OTC) | Brompheniramine Maleate | Phenylpropanola-HCl | |
| Bromphen TD (℞) | Bromphenira-mine Maleate | Phenylpropanola-mine HCl, Phenylephrine HCl | |
| Carbodec (℞) | Carbinoxamine Maleate | Pseudoephedrine HCl | |
| Cardec-S (℞) | Carbinoxamine Maleate | Pseudoephedrine HCl | |
| Cheracol Sinus (OTC) | Dexbrompheniramine Maleate | Pseudoephedrine Sulfate | |
| Children's Tylenol Cold (OTC) | Methscopolamine Nitrate | Pseudoephedrine HCl | Acetaminophen |
| Chlor-Trimeton Sinus (OTC) | Chlorpheniramine Maleate | Phenylpropanola-mine HCl | Acetaminophen |
| Claritin-D (℞) | Loratadine | Pseudoephedrine HCl | |
| Codimal LA (℞) | Chlorpheniramine Maleate | Pseudoephedrine HCl | |
| Comhist (℞) | Chlorpheniramine Maleate, Phenyltoloxamine Citrate | Phenylephrine HCl | |

Respiratory

Numerous combination products are available both by prescription and over-the-counter for respiratory conditions. Often a product may either contain ingredients not needed or the wrong strength of an ingredient that is needed. It is advisable to avoid "shotgun" therapy with combination products unless needed. Using a multiple-ingredient product when not necessary can increase the risk for side effects and drug interactions.

The following tables identify commonly used products with the ingredients contained in each. Many common brand names formerly associated with one ingredient may have several different formulations on the market. It is important to identify the ingredients in a product. Detailed information on all the ingredients included in this table is provided elsewhere in the text.

**INDICATION** These products are generally used for runny noses, head congestion, sinus headaches, and sneezing.

**BANNED SUBSTANCES** NCAA and/or USOC may list some of these substances as banned for athletes to use.

| Brand Name | Antihistamine | Decongestant | Analgesic/Other |
|---|---|---|---|
| Comhist LA (℞) | Chlorpheniramine Maleate, Phenyltoloxamine Citrate | Phenylephrine HCl | |
| Comtrex Allergy-Sinus (OTC) | Methscopolamine Nitrate | Pseudoephedrine HCl | Acetaminophen |
| Congestant (OTC) | Chlorpheniramine Maleate | | Acetaminophen |
| Contac (OTC) | Chlorpheniramine Maleate | Phenylpropanolamine HCl | |
| Coricidin (OTC) | Chlorpheniramine Maleate | | Acetaminophen |
| Coricidin D (OTC) | Chlorpheniramine Maleate | Phenylpropanolamine HCl | Acetaminophen |
| Dallergy D (OTC) | Chlorpheniramine Maleate | Phenylephrine HCl | |
| Dallergy (℞) | Chlorpheniramine Maleate | Phenylpropanolamine HCl | Methscopolamine Nitrate |
| Dallergy-JR (℞) | Brompheniramine Maleate | Pseudoephedrine HCl | |
| Deconamine SR (℞) | Chlorpheniramine Maleate | Pseudoephedrine HCl | |
| Demazin (OTC) | Chlorpheniramine Maleate | Phenylpropanolamine HCl | |

Numerous combination products are available both by prescription and over-the-counter for respiratory conditions. Often a product may either contain ingredients not needed or the wrong strength of an ingredient that is needed. It is advisable to avoid "shotgun" therapy with combination products unless needed. Using a multiple-ingredient product when not necessary can increase the risk for side effects and drug interactions.

The following tables identify commonly used products with the ingredients contained in each. Many common brand names formerly associated with one ingredient may have several different formulations on the market. It is important to identify the ingredients in a product. Detailed information on all the ingredients included in this table is provided elsewhere in the text.

**INDICATION** These products are generally used for runny noses, head congestion, sinus headaches, and sneezing.

**BANNED SUBSTANCES** NCAA and/or USOC may list some of these substances as banned for athletes to use.

| Brand Name | Antihistamine | Decongestant | Analgesic/Other |
|---|---|---|---|
| Dimetane De-congestant | Brompheniramine Maleate | Phenylephrine HCI | |
| Dimetapp (OTC) | Brompheniramine Maleate | Phenylpropanola-mine HCI | |
| Dimetapp Sinus (OTC) | | Pseudoephedrine HCI | Ibuprofen |
| Disophrol (OTC) | Dexbromphenira-mine Maleate | Pseudoephedrine Sulfate | |
| Dristan Cold (OTC) | Brompheniramine Maleate | Phenylephrine HCI | Acetaminophen |
| Dristan Cold Multi-Symptom Formula (OTC) | Chlorpheniramine Maleate | Phenylephrine HCI | Acetaminophen |
| Dristan Allergy (OTC) | Brompheniramine Maleate | Pseudoephedrine HCI | |
| Drixoral Cold & Allergy (OTC) | Dexbromphenira-mine Maleate | Pseudoephedrine Sulfate | |
| Drixoral (OTC) | Dexbromphenira-mine Maleate | Pseudoephedrine Sulfate | Acetaminophen |
| Dura-Vent/DA (℞) | Chlorpheniramine Maleate | Phenylpropanola-mine HCI | Methscopolamine Nitrate |
| Dura-Vent A (℞) | Chlorpheniramine Maleate | Phenylpropanola-mine HCI | |
| Endafed (℞) | Brompheniramine Maleate | Pseudoephedrine HCI | |

Numerous combination products are available both by prescription and over-the-counter for respiratory conditions. Often a product may either contain ingredients not needed or the wrong strength of an ingredient that is needed. It is advisable to avoid "shotgun" therapy with combination products unless needed. Using a multiple-ingredient product when not necessary can increase the risk for side effects and drug interactions.

The following tables identify commonly used products with the ingredients contained in each. Many common brand names formerly associated with one ingredient may have several different formulations on the market. It is important to identify the ingredients in a product. Detailed information on all the ingredients included in this table is provided elsewhere in the text.

**INDICATION** These products are generally used for runny noses, head congestion, sinus headaches, and sneezing.

**BANNED SUBSTANCES** NCAA and/or USOC may list some of these substances as banned for athletes to use.

| Brand Name | Antihistamine | Decongestant | Analgesic/Other |
|------------|---------------|--------------|-----------------|
| Extendryl SR (℞) | Chlorpheniramine Maleate | Phenylpropanola-mine HCl | Methscopolamine Nitrate |
| Extendryl JR (℞) | Chlorpheniramine Maleate | Phenylephrine HCl | |
| Fedahist (OTC) | Chlorpheniramine Maleate | Pseudoephedrine HCl | |
| Histalet Forte (℞) | Chlorpheniramine Maleate, Pyrilamine Maleate | Phenylpropanola-mine HCl, Phenylephrine HCl | |
| Histalet (℞) | Chlorpheniramine Maleate | Pseudoephedrine HCl | |
| Isoclor (OTC) | Chlorpheniramine Maleate | Pseudoephedrine HCl | |
| Lodrane LD (℞) | Brompheniramine Maleate | Pseudoephedrine HCl | |
| Mescolor (℞) | Chlorpheniramine Maleate | Pseudoephedrine HCl | Methscopolamine Nitrate |
| Naldecon (℞) | Chlorpheniramine Maleate, Phenylto-loxamine Citrate | Phenylpropanola-mine HCl, Phenylephrine HCl | |
| Nalgest (℞) | Chlorpheniramine Maleate, Phenylto-loxamine Citrate | Phenylpropanola-mine HCl, Phenylephrine HCl | |

Numerous combination products are available both by prescription and over-the-counter for respiratory conditions. Often a product may either contain ingredients not needed or the wrong strength of an ingredient that is needed. It is advisable to avoid "shotgun" therapy with combination products unless needed. Using a multiple-ingredient product when not necessary can increase the risk for side effects and drug interactions.

The following tables identify commonly used products with the ingredients contained in each. Many common brand names formerly associated with one ingredient may have several different formulations on the market. It is important to identify the ingredients in a product. Detailed information on all the ingredients included in this table is provided elsewhere in the text.

**INDICATION** These products are generally used for runny noses, head congestion, sinus headaches, and sneezing.

**BANNED SUBSTANCES** NCAA and/or USOC may list some of these substances as banned for athletes to use.

| Brand Name | Antihistamine | Decongestant | Analgesic/Other |
|---|---|---|---|
| *Nolamine* (℞) | Chlorpheniramine Maleate, Phenindamine Tartrate | Phenylephrine HCl | |
| *Novafed A* (℞) | Chlorpheniramine Maleate | Pseudoephedrine HCl | |
| *Novahistine* Elixir (OTC) | Chlorpheniramine Maleate | Phenylephrine HCl | |
| *Ornade* (℞) | Chlorpheniramine Maleate | Phenylpropanolamine HCl | |
| *Ornex* (OTC) | | Pseudoephedrine HCl | Acetaminophen |
| *Pedia-Care Cold-Allergy* (OTC) | Chlorpheniramine Maleate | Pseudoephedrine HCl | |
| *Percogesic* (OTC) | Phenyltoloxamine Citrate | | Acetaminophen |
| *Phenate* (℞) | Chlorpheniramine Maleate | Phenylpropanolamine HCl | Acetaminophen |
| *Phenchlor SHA* (℞) | Chlorpheniramine Maleate | Phenylpropanolamine HCl, Phenylephrine HCl | Belladonna Alkaloids |
| *Phenergan VC* (℞) | Promethazine HCl | Phenylephrine HCl | |
| *Poly-Histine-D* (℞) | Phenyltoloxamine Citrate, Pyrilamine Maleate, Pheniramine Maleate | Phenylephrine HCl | |

Numerous combination products are available both by prescription and over-the-counter for respiratory conditions. Often a product may either contain ingredients not needed or the wrong strength of an ingredient that is needed. It is advisable to avoid "shotgun" therapy with combination products unless needed. Using a multiple-ingredient product when not necessary can increase the risk for side effects and drug interactions.

The following tables identify commonly used products with the ingredients contained in each. Many common brand names formerly associated with one ingredient may have several different formulations on the market. It is important to identify the ingredients in a product. Detailed information on all the ingredients included in this table is provided elsewhere in the text.

**INDICATION** These products are generally used for runny noses, head congestion, sinus headaches, and sneezing.

**BANNED SUBSTANCES** NCAA and/or USOC may list some of these substances as banned for athletes to use.

| Brand Name | Antihistamine | Decongestant | Analgesic/Other |
|---|---|---|---|
| Prehist (℞) | Chlorpheniramine Maleate | Phenylephrine HCl | |
| Prometh VC (℞) | Promethazine HCl | Phenylephrine HCl | |
| R-Tannate (℞) | Chlorpheniramine Maleate, Pyrilamine Tannate | Phenylephrine Tannate | |
| Resaid (℞) | Chlorpheniramine Maleate | Phenylpropanola-mine HCl | |
| Rondec TR (℞) | Carbinoxamine Maleate | Pseudoephedrine HCl | |
| Ru-Tuss (℞) | Chlorpheniramine Maleate | Phenylpropanola-mine HCl, Phenylephrine HCl | Belladonna Alkaloids |
| Ru-Tuss II (℞) | Chlorpheniramine Maleate | Phenylpropanola-mine HCl | |
| Rynatan (℞) | Chlorpheniramine Maleate, Pyrilamine Tannate | Phenylephrine Tannate | |
| Seldane-D (℞) | Terfenadine | Pseudoephedrine HCl | |
| Sinarest (OTC) | Methscopolamine Nitrate | Pseudoephedrine HCl | Acetaminophen |
| Sine-Aid IB (OTC) | | Pseudoephedrine HCl | Ibuprofen |

Numerous combination products are available both by prescription and over-the-counter for respiratory conditions. Often a product may either contain ingredients not needed or the wrong strength of an ingredient that is needed. It is advisable to avoid "shotgun" therapy with combination products unless needed. Using a multiple-ingredient product when not necessary can increase the risk for side effects and drug interactions.

The following tables identify commonly used products with the ingredients contained in each. Many common brand names formerly associated with one ingredient may have several different formulations on the market. It is important to identify the ingredients in a product. Detailed information on all the ingredients included in this table is provided elsewhere in the text.

**INDICATION** These products are generally used for runny noses, head congestion, sinus headaches, and sneezing.

**BANNED SUBSTANCES** NCAA and/or USOC may list some of these substances as banned for athletes to use.

| Brand Name | Antihistamine | Decongestant | Analgesic/Other |
|---|---|---|---|
| Sine-Off (OTC) | Methscopolamine Nitrate | Pseudoephedrine HCl | Acetaminophen |
| Singlet (OTC) | Methscopolamine Nitrate | Pseudoephedrine HCl | Acetaminophen |
| Sinulin (OTC) | Chlorpheniramine Maleate | Phenylpropanolamine HCl | Acetaminophen |
| Sinus-Relief (OTC) | | Pseudoephedrine HCl | Acetaminophen |
| Sinutab w/o Drowsiness (OTC) | | Pseudoephedrine HCl | Acetaminophen |
| St. Joseph Cold (OTC) | | Phenylpropanolamine HCl | Acetaminophen |
| Sudafed Plus (OTC) | Chlorpheniramine Maleate | Pseudoephedrine HCl | |
| Tavist-D (OTC) | Clemastine Fumarate | Phenylpropanolamine HCl | |
| Temazin (OTC) | Chlorpheniramine Maleate | Phenylpropanolamine HCl | |
| TheraFlu and Cold Powder (OTC) | Methscopolamine Nitrate | Pseudoephedrine HCl | Acetaminophen |
| Triaminic (OTC) | Chlorpheniramine Maleate | Phenylpropanolamine HCl | |
| Triaminicin (OTC) | Chlorpheniramine Maleate | Phenylpropanolamine HCl | Acetaminophen |

Respiratory

Numerous combination products are available both by prescription and over-the-counter for respiratory conditions. Often a product may either contain ingredients not needed or the wrong strength of an ingredient that is needed. It is advisable to avoid "shotgun" therapy with combination products unless needed. Using a multiple-ingredient product when not necessary can increase the risk for side effects and drug interactions.

The following tables identify commonly used products with the ingredients contained in each. Many common brand names formerly associated with one ingredient may have several different formulations on the market. It is important to identify the ingredients in a product. Detailed information on all the ingredients included in this table is provided elsewhere in the text.

**INDICATION** These products are generally used for runny noses, head congestion, sinus headaches, and sneezing.

**BANNED SUBSTANCES** NCAA and/or USOC may list some of these substances as banned for athletes to use.

| Brand Name | Antihistamine | Decongestant | Analgesic/Other |
|------------|---------------|--------------|-----------------|
| Trifed (OTC) | Triprolidine HCl | Pseudoephedrine HCl | |
| Trinalin Repetabs (℞) | Azatadine Maleate | Pseudoephedrine Sulfate | |
| Triotann (℞) | Chlorpheniramine Maleate, Pyrilamine Tannate | Phenylephrine Tannate | |
| Triprolidine HCl-Phen-Chlor (℞) | Chlorpheniramine Maleate, Phenyltoloxamine Citrate | Phenylpropanolamine HCl, Phenylephrine HCl | |
| Tylenol Flu Nighttime (OTC) | Diphenhydramine HCl | Pseudoephedrine HCl | Acetaminophen |
| Tylenol PM (OTC) | Diphenhydramine HCl | | Acetaminophen |
| ULTRAbrom PD (℞) | Brompheniramine Maleate | Pseudoephedrine HCl | |
| Vanex Forte (℞) | Chlorpheniramine Maleate, Pyrilamine Maleate | Phenylpropanolamine HCl, Phenylephrine HCl | |

# Cardiovascular Agents

## Alpha-1-Adrenergic Blockers

**ACTION** Alpha-1-adrenergic blocking agents dilate both veins and arteries to reduce resistance against the blood flow, lowering blood pressure. This generally has no effect on the heart rate and will lower both resting and exercising blood pressure.

**INDICATION** Used to lower high blood pressure.

| Generic Name<br>*Brand Name* | Side Effects | Warnings | Dosing | Notes |
|---|---|---|---|---|
| **Doxazosin**<br>*Cardura* tablet<br>(℞) | Nausea, indigestion, depression, shortness of breath, sweating, flushing, blurred vision, dizziness, drowsiness. | Use caution when rising from a sitting or lying position. | Take without regard for food. | Also used to improve symptoms of benign prostatic hyperplasia. |
| **Prazosin**<br>*Minipres* capsule<br>(℞) | Nausea, indigestion, depression, shortness of breath, sweating, flushing, blurred vision, dizziness, drowsiness. | Use caution when rising from a sitting or lying position. | Take without regard for food. | |
| **Tamsulosin**<br>*Flomax* capsule<br>(℞) | Dizziness, rhinitis, infection, syncope. | | | Only used to improve symptoms of benign prostatic hyperplasia. Not effective for reducing blood pressure. |
| **Terazosin**<br>*Hytrin* tablet<br>or capsule (℞) | Nausea, indigestion, depression, shortness of breath, sweating, flushing, blurred vision, dizziness, or drowsiness. | Use caution when rising from a sitting or lying position. | Take without regard for food. | Also used to improve symptoms of benign prostatic hyperplasia. |

## Alpha-1-Agonist

**ACTION** Activates alpha-adrenergic receptors producing an increase in vascular tone and elevation of blood pressure.

**INDICATION** Used to increase standing blood pressure.

| Generic Name<br>Brand Name | Side Effects | Warnings | Dosing | Notes |
|---|---|---|---|---|
| **Midodrine HCl**<br>ProAmatine tablet<br>(℞) | Supine hypertension, pruritus, goose bumps, chills, urinary urge, urinary frequency. | Do not take with decongestants found in cough and cold medications, or with diet-aid products that may enhance the effect of midodrine. | Do not take within 4 hours of bedtime. | |

## Angiotensin-Converting Enzyme Inhibitors

**ACTION** Angiotensin-converting enzyme (ACE) inhibitors lower blood pressure by blocking enzymes that constrict blood vessels, increase blood pressure, and cause sodium retention. Some ACE inhibitors may also increase the heart's ability to pump blood. This generally has no effect on the heart rate and lowers both resting and exercising blood pressure.

**INDICATION** Used to lower high blood pressure either alone or in combination with other blood pressure medications.

| Generic Name<br>Brand Name | Side Effects | Warnings | Dosing | Notes |
|---|---|---|---|---|
| **Benazepril HCl**<br>Lotensin tablet<br>(℞) | Nausea, diarrhea, constipation, depression, chest pain, shortness of breath, edema. | Avoid cough, cold, or allergy medications except on professional recommendation. | May take without regard for food. | |

**ACTION** Angiotensin-converting enzyme (ACE) inhibitors lower blood pressure by blocking enzymes that constrict blood vessels, increase blood pressure, and cause sodium retention. Some ACE inhibitors may also increase the heart's ability to pump blood. This generally has no effect on the heart rate and lowers both resting and exercising blood pressure.

**INDICATION** Used to lower high blood pressure either alone or in combination with other blood pressure medications.

| Generic Name<br>Brand Name | Side Effects | Warnings | Dosing | Notes |
|---|---|---|---|---|
| **Captopril**<br>*Capoten* tablet<br>(℞) | Nausea, diarrhea, constipation, depression, chest pain, shortness of breath, edema. | Avoid cough, cold, or allergy medications except on professional recommendation. | Take 1 hour before or 2 hours after meals. | Used to treat certain types of heart failure and diabetic nephropathy. |
| **Enalapril Maleate**<br>*Vasotec* tablet (℞) | Nausea, diarrhea, constipation, depression, chest pain, shortness of breath, edema. | Avoid cough, cold, or allergy medications except on professional recommendation. | May take without regard to food. | Used to treat certain types of heart failure. |
| **Fosinopril Sodium**<br>*Monopril* tablet (℞) | Nausea, diarrhea, constipation, depression, chest pain, shortness of breath, edema. | Avoid cough, cold, or allergy medications except on professional recommendation. | May take without regard to food. | |
| **Lisinopril**<br>*Prinivil, Zestril* tablet (℞) | Nausea, diarrhea, constipation, depression, chest pain, shortness of breath, edema. | Avoid cough, cold, or allergy medications except on professional recommendation. | May take without regard to food. | Used to treat certain types of heart failure. |
| **Moexipril HCl**<br>*Univasc* tablet (℞) | Nausea, diarrhea, constipation, depression, chest pain, shortness of breath, edema. | Avoid cough, cold, or allergy medications except on professional recommendation. | Take 1 hour before or 2 hours after meals. | Used to treat certain types of heart failure. |

Cardiovascular

**ACTION** Angiotensin-converting enzyme (ACE) inhibitors lower blood pressure by blocking enzymes that constrict blood vessels, increase blood pressure, and cause sodium retention. Some ACE inhibitors may also increase the heart's ability to pump blood. This generally has no effect on the heart rate and lowers both resting and exercising blood pressure.

**INDICATION** Used to lower high blood pressure either alone or in combination with other blood pressure medications.

| Generic Name<br>*Brand Name* | Side Effects | Warnings | Dosing | Notes |
|---|---|---|---|---|
| **Quinapril HCl**<br>*Accupril* tablet (℞) | Nausea, diarrhea, constipation, depression, chest pain, shortness of breath, edema. | Avoid cough, cold, or allergy medications except on professional recommendation. | Take 1 hour before or 2 hours after meals. | Used to treat certain types of heart failure. |
| **Ramipril**<br>*Altace* capsule (℞) | Nausea, diarrhea, constipation, depression, chest pain, shortness of breath, edema. | Avoid cough, cold, or allergy medications except on professional recommendation. | May take without regard to food. | |
| **Trandolapril**<br>*Mavik* tablet (℞) | Nausea, vomiting, diarrhea, headache, dizziness, fatigue. | Avoid cough, cold, or allergy medications except on professional recommendation. | May take without regard for food. | |

## Antianginal Agents

**ACTION** Antianginal agents relax blood vessels, which allows them to dilate and carry more blood flow. This increased blood flow reduces the workload of the heart and reduces the oxygen demand of the heart. These agents may increase heart rate, lower blood pressure, and thus may increase exercise capacity or may have no affect at all.

**INDICATION** Used to treat and prevent angina (chest pain) attacks. These drugs may be used before an event that could precipitate an angina attack. They may also be used to treat congestive heart failure associated with heart attacks.

| Generic Name<br>*Brand Name* | Side Effects | Warnings | Dosing | Notes |
|---|---|---|---|---|
| **Amyl Nitrate**<br>*Amyl Nitrate*<br>Inhalant (℞) | Lightheadedness, dizziness, headaches, euphoria. | Avoid alcohol. Use only when lying down. Highly flammable, use in a well-ventilated area. | | Amyl nitrate is abused for sexual stimulation. |
| **Erythrityl Tetranitrate**<br>*Cardilate* tablet (℞) | Headaches, faintness, flushing, nausea, vomiting. | Avoid alcohol. | Take on an empty stomach with a glass of water. | Tablets may be dissolved under the tongue, but do not chew or crush tablet. |
| **Isosorbide Dinitrate**<br>*Isordil,*<br>*Sorbitrate* tablet (℞)<br>*Dilatrate-SR,*<br>*Iso-BID, Isordil*<br>*Tembids* capsule (℞) | Headaches, faintness, flushing, nausea, vomiting. | Avoid alcohol. | Take on an empty stomach with a glass of water. | Some tablets may be dissolved under the tongue, but do not chew or crush tablet. Some tablets and capsules are sustained-release and should be swallowed whole. |
| **Isosorbide Mononitrate**<br>*Ismo, Monoket,*<br>*Imdur* tablet (℞) | Headaches, faintness, flushing, nausea, vomiting. | Avoid alcohol. | Take on an empty stomach with a glass of water. | |

Cardiovascular

**ACTION** Antianginal agents relax blood vessels, which allows them to dilate and carry more blood flow. This increased blood flow reduces the workload of the heart and reduces the oxygen demand of the heart. These agents may increase heart rate, lower blood pressure, and thus may increase exercise capacity or may have no affect at all.

**INDICATION** Used to treat and prevent angina (chest pain) attacks. These drugs may be used before an event that could precipitate an angina attack. They may also be used to treat congestive heart failure associated with heart attacks.

| Generic Name<br>*Brand Name* | Side Effects | Warnings | Dosing | Notes |
|---|---|---|---|---|
| **Nitroglycerin**<br>*Nitrostat*<br>sublingual tablet (℞)<br>*Nitro-Bid, Nitroglyn*<br>sustained-release capsule (℞)<br>*Nitro-Bid, Nitrol*<br>topical ointment (℞)<br>*Nitrolingual* spray (℞)<br>*Minitran, Nitro-Dur, Transderm-Nitro, Deponit* trans-dermal patch (℞) | Headaches, faint-ness, flushing, nausea, vomit-ing, contact dermatitis. | Avoid alcohol. Tolerance to nitroglycerin may develop requiring dosage adjust-ments. | Take on an empty stomach with a glass of water. | Patches and sustained-release products are not for the immediate relief of chest pain. Each dosage form has special precautions. Con-sult a physician or pharmacist. Used patches should be dis-posed of pro-perly away from children and pets. |

## Antiarrhythmic Agents

**ACTION** Antiarrhythmic agents correct and prevent the occurrence of various types of irregular heart rhythms that can lead to life-threatening situations. All antiarrhythmics may affect heart rate and blood pressure, and thus may increase, decrease, or have no effect on exercise capacity.

**INDICATION** Used to treat different types of irregular heartbeats.

| Generic Name<br>*Brand Name* | Side Effects | Warnings | Dosing | Notes |
|---|---|---|---|---|
| **Amiodarone**<br>*Cordarone* tablet (℞) | Blurred vision, nausea, tremors, fatigue, short-ness of breath, edema. | Sensitivity to sunlight may occur. Notify a doctor if visual effects are ex-perienced. | Take with meals. | Generally used when other therapies fail to work. |

**ACTION** Antiarrhythmic agents correct and prevent the occurrence of various types of irregular heart rhythms that can lead to life-threatening situations. All antiarrhythmics may affect heart rate and blood pressure, and thus may increase, decrease, or have no effect on exercise capacity.

**INDICATION** Used to treat different types of irregular heartbeats.

| Generic Name<br>*Brand Name* | Side Effects | Warnings | Dosing | Notes |
|---|---|---|---|---|
| **Disopyramide**<br>*Norpace* capsule (℞)<br>*Norpace CR* extended-release capsule (℞) | Constipation, nausea, head-ache, nervous-ness, chest pain, itching, short-ness of breath, edema. | Contact a doctor if dry mouth, dizziness, consti-pation, or blurred vision continue. | | May be used for certain types of rapid heart rates. |
| **Flecainide Acetate**<br>*Tambocor* tablet (℞) | Nausea, vomit-ing, constipation, dizziness, head-ache, nervous-ness, depression, chest pain, flush-ing, edema, and blurred vision. | Serious heart-beat disturbances can occur from missing a dose. | | This drug may require routine blood tests to monitor drug levels. |
| **Mexiletine**<br>*Mexitil* capsule (℞) | Nausea, heart-burn, constipa-tion, headache, nervousness, blurred vision, weakness, chest pain. | Avoid diet changes that could drastically alter the pH of your urine. If side effects per-sist, contact a physician. | Take with food or an antacid. | May be used in association with diabetic neu-ropathy and to reduce irregular heartbeats during a heart attack. |
| **Moricizine**<br>*Ethmozine* tablet (℞) | Nausea, vomit-ing, dizziness, drowsiness, headache, chest pain, asthma, cough, urinary retention, and blurred vision. | Contact a doctor if chest pain, fever, or irregular heartbeat de-velops. | Serious heart-beat disturbances can occur from missing a dose. | |
| **Procainamide**<br>*Pronestyl* capsule, tablet (℞)<br>*Pronestyl-SR, Procan SR* sustained-release capsule (℞) | Appetite loss, nausea, depres-sion, dizziness, bitter taste. | Notify a doctor if joint pain, fever, easy bruising, wheezing, diar-rhea, or dark urine is ex-perienced. | | Do not break or chew sustained-release tablets |

**ACTION** Antiarrhythmic agents correct and prevent the occurrence of various types of irregular heart rhythms that can lead to life-threatening situations. All antiarrhythmics may affect heart rate and blood pressure, and thus may increase, decrease, or have no effect on exercise capacity.

**INDICATION** Used to treat different types of irregular heartbeats.

| Generic Name<br>*Brand Name* | Side Effects | Warnings | Dosing | Notes |
|---|---|---|---|---|
| **Propafenone HCl**<br>*Rythmol* tablet (℞) | Nausea, vomiting, dizziness, drowsiness, headache, chest pain, blurred vision. | Watch for signs of toxicity such as excessive drowsiness, slowed heart rate, or lowered blood pressure. | | May be used for Wolff-Parkinson-White syndrome. |
| **Quinidine Gluconate**<br>*Quinaglute, Quinalan* sustained-release tablet (℞) | Nausea, vomiting, dizziness, headache, confusion, rash, blurred vision, or fainting. | Notify a doctor if ringing in the ears, visual disturbances, or difficult breathing is experienced. | Take with food; may cause stomach upset. | Used to treat some types of malaria when a rapid effect is desired. Do not crush tablets. |
| **Quinidine Polygalacturonate**<br>*Cardioquin* tablet (℞) | Nausea, vomiting, dizziness, headache, confusion, rash, blurred vision, or fainting. | Notify a doctor if ringing in the ears, visual disturbances, or difficult breathing is experienced. | Take with food; may cause stomach upset. | Used to treat some types of malaria when a rapid effect is desired. |
| **Quinidine Sulfate**<br>*Quinora* tablet (℞)<br>*Quinidex Extentab* sustained-release tablet (℞) | Nausea, vomiting, dizziness, headache, confusion, rash, blurred vision, or fainting. | Notify a doctor if ringing in the ears, visual disturbances, or difficult breathing is experienced. | Take with food; may cause stomach upset. | Used to treat some types of malaria when a rapid effect is desired. Do not chew or crush sustained-release tablet. |
| **Tocainide**<br>*Tonocard* tablet (℞) | Nausea, vomiting, dizziness, vertigo, blurred vision, hearing loss, or muscle pain. | Notify a doctor if painful breathing, easy bruising, soreness in the mouth, or tremors are experienced. | May cause drowsiness. | May be used to treat myotonic dystrophy and trigeminal neuralgia. |

# Antihyperlipidemics

**ACTION** High levels of cholesterol and triglycerides may block blood vessels and increase the risk of heart or blood vessel disease. These medications either increase the rate of removal of cholesterol from the blood or reduce the production of certain types of cholesterol by the body.

**INDICATION** As an adjunct to diet and exercise, antihyperlipidemics are used to lower high levels of cholesterol and triglycerides in the blood.

| Generic Name<br>Brand Name | Side Effects | Warnings | Dosing | Notes |
|---|---|---|---|---|
| **Atorvastatin Calcium**<br>*Lipitor* tablet (R) | Myalgia, head-ache, rash, fla-tulence, dyspep-sia, infection, abdominal pain. | Contact a physi-cian if symptoms of unexplained muscle pain, tenderness, weakness, or fever occur. | Can be taken with or without food. | |
| **Cerivastatin Sodium**<br>*Baycol* (R) | Rhinitis, pharyn-gitis, headache. | | Take with or without food. | |
| **Cholestyramine**<br>*Cholybar, Questran, Prevalite* bar, powder (R) | Constipation, gas, nausea, heartburn, head-ache, itching, or appetite loss. | | Take before meals. Powders to be mixed with liquids before taking. | Has been used to treat certain toxicities by binding to the toxin in the digestive tract. Most effective when used with a diet low in cholesterol and saturated fats. |
| **Clofibrate**<br>*Atromid-S* capsule (R) | Stomach pain, nausea, diarrhea, fatigue, head-ache, itching, hair loss, swell-ing, or appetite loss. | Notify a doctor if chest pain, short-ness of breath, stomach pain, or blood in the urine occurs. | If upset stomach occurs, take with food. | Most effective when used with a diet low in cholesterol and saturated fats. |

Cardiovascular

**ACTION** High levels of cholesterol and triglycerides may block blood vessels and increase the risk of heart or blood vessel disease. These medications either increase the rate of removal of cholesterol from the blood or reduce the production of certain types of cholesterol by the body.

**INDICATION** As an adjunct to diet and exercise, antihyperlipidemics are used to lower high levels of cholesterol and triglycerides in the blood.

| Generic Name Brand Name | Side Effects | Warnings | Dosing | Notes |
|---|---|---|---|---|
| **Colestipol HCL** *Colestid* powder (℞) | Constipation, gas, nausea, heartburn, headache, itching, or appetite loss. | | Take before meals. Powders to be mixed with liquids before taking. | Has been used to treat certain toxicities by binding to the toxin in the digestive tract. Most effective when used with a diet low in cholesterol and saturated fats. |
| **Fluvastatin Sodium** *Lescol* capsule (℞) | Stomach pain, nausea, constipation, diarrhea, headache, itching, blurred vision. | | Take with the evening meal. | Most effective when used with exercise and a diet low in cholesterol and saturated fats. |
| **Gemfibrozil** *Lopid, Gemcor* tablet (℞) | Indigestion, stomach pain, nausea, diarrhea, fatigue, headache, itching, dizziness, vertigo, blurred vision. | Avoid alcohol while taking this medicine. Notify a doctor if you ongoing abdominal pain, diarrhea, nausea, or vomiting occurs. | Take 30 minutes before meals. | Most effective when used with a diet low in cholesterol and saturated fats. |

**ACTION** High levels of cholesterol and triglycerides may block blood vessels and increase the risk of heart or blood vessel disease. These medications either increase the rate of removal of cholesterol from the blood or reduce the production of certain types of cholesterol by the body.

**INDICATION** As an adjunct to diet and exercise, antihyperlipidemics are used to lower high levels of cholesterol and triglycerides in the blood.

| Generic Name Brand Name | Side Effects | Warnings | Dosing | Notes |
|---|---|---|---|---|
| **Lovastatin** *Mevacor* tablet (℞) | Stomach pain, nausea, constipation, diarrhea, headache, itching, blurred vision. | | Take with the evening meal. | May also be used for high cholesterol due to diabetes, certain kidney diseases, and hereditary disorders. Most effective when used with exercise and a diet low in cholesterol and saturated fats. |
| **Pravastatin Sodium** *Pravachol* tablet (℞) | Stomach pain, nausea, constipation, diarrhea, headache, itching, blurred vision. | | Take once daily at bedtime without regard to meals. | May also be used for high cholesterol due to diabetes, certain kidney diseases, and hereditary disorders. Most effective when used with exercise and a diet low in cholesterol and saturated fats. |
| **Probucol** *Lorelco* tablet (℞) | Stomach pain, nausea, constipation, diarrhea, headache, itching, blurred vision. | | Take with meals. | Most effective when used with exercise and a diet low in cholesterol and saturated fats. |

Cardiovascular

**ACTION** High levels of cholesterol and triglycerides may block blood vessels and increase the risk of heart or blood vessel disease. These medications either increase the rate of removal of cholesterol from the blood or reduce the production of certain types of cholesterol by the body.

**INDICATION** As an adjunct to diet and exercise, antihyperlipidemics are used to lower high levels of cholesterol and triglycerides in the blood.

| Generic Name<br>*Brand Name* | Side Effects | Warnings | Dosing | Notes |
|---|---|---|---|---|
| **Simvastatin**<br>*Zocor* tablet (℞) | Stomach pain, nausea, constipation, diarrhea, headache, itching, blurred vision. | | Take in the evening without regard to meals. | May also be used for high cholesterol due to diabetes, certain kidney diseases, and hereditary disorders. Most effective when used with exercise and a diet low in cholesterol and saturated fats. |

# Beta-Adrenergic Blocking Agents

**ACTION** Beta blockers slow the heart rate, reduce output of the heart at rest and during exercise, and slow conduction of nerve impulses in the heart and other organs. This generally reduces both the resting and exercising heart rates and will lower both resting and exercising blood pressures. These drugs may increase exercise capacity in patients with angina. These products may mask signs of low blood sugar in diabetics. Inform the doctor or dentist of use before any type of surgery.

**INDICATION** Used to lower high blood pressure either alone or in combination with other blood pressure medications.

**BANNED SUBSTANCES** NCAA and/or USOC may list some of these substances as banned for athletes to use.

| Generic Name<br>*Brand Name* | Side Effects | Warnings | Dosing | Notes |
|---|---|---|---|---|
| **Acebutolol**<br>*Sectral* capsule (℞) | Nausea, vomiting, depression, anxiety, chest pain, shortness of breath, swelling, flushing, aching, eye problems, dry mouth. | | May be taken without regard to meals. | May also be used to treat irregular heartbeats. |
| **Atenolol**<br>*Tenormin* tablet (℞) | Nausea, vomiting, depression, anxiety, chest pain, shortness of breath, swelling, flushing, aching, eye problems, dry mouth. | | May be taken without regard to meals. | May also be used to treat angina, heart attack, stage fright, and to prevent migraine headaches. |
| **Betaxolol HCl**<br>*Kerlone* tablet (℞) | Nausea, vomiting, depression, anxiety, chest pain, shortness of breath, swelling, flushing, aching, eye problems, dry mouth. | Consult with a health professional before taking with nasal decongestants or other cough and cold products. | | |

Cardiovascular

**ACTION** Beta blockers slow the heart rate, reduce output of the heart at rest and during exercise, and slow conduction of nerve impulses in the heart and other organs. This generally reduces both the resting and exercising heart rates and will lower both resting and exercising blood pressures. These drugs may increase exercise capacity in patients with angina. These products may mask signs of low blood sugar in diabetics. Inform the doctor or dentist of use before any type of surgery.

**INDICATION** Used to lower high blood pressure either alone or in combination with other blood pressure medications.

**BANNED SUBSTANCES** NCAA and/or USOC may list some of these substances as banned for athletes to use.

| Generic Name<br>*Brand Name* | Side Effects | Warnings | Dosing | Notes |
|---|---|---|---|---|
| **Bisoprolol Fumarate**<br>*Zebeta* tablet (℞) | Nausea, vomiting, depression, anxiety, chest pain, shortness of breath, swelling, flushing, aching, eye problems, dry mouth. | | May be taken without regard to meals. | |
| **Carteolol HCl**<br>*Cartrol* tablet (℞) | Nausea, vomiting, depression, anxiety, chest pain, shortness of breath, swelling, flushing, aching, eye problems, dry mouth. | | May be taken without regard to meals. | May also be used to treat angina. |
| **Metoprolol Succinate**<br>*Toprol XL* extended-release tablet (℞) | Nausea, vomiting, depression, anxiety, chest pain, shortness of breath, swelling, flushing, aching, eye problems, dry mouth. | Do not crush or chew tablet. | Take consistently with or immediately following meals. | May also be used to treat angina. |
| **Metoprolol Tartrate**<br>*Lopressor* tablet (℞) | Nausea, vomiting, depression, anxiety, chest pain, shortness of breath, swelling, flushing, aching, eye problems, dry mouth. | | Take consistently with or without food at the same time each day. | May also be used to treat angina, heart attacks, tremors, and to prevent migraines. |

**ACTION** Beta blockers slow the heart rate, reduce output of the heart at rest and during exercise, and slow conduction of nerve impulses in the heart and other organs. This generally reduces both the resting and exercising heart rates and will lower both resting and exercising blood pressures. These drugs may increase exercise capacity in patients with angina. These products may mask signs of low blood sugar in diabetics. Inform the doctor or dentist of use before any type of surgery.

**INDICATION** Used to lower high blood pressure either alone or in combination with other blood pressure medications.

**BANNED SUBSTANCES** NCAA and/or USOC may list some of these substances as banned for athletes to use.

| Generic Name<br>*Brand Name* | Side Effects | Warnings | Dosing | Notes |
|---|---|---|---|---|
| **Nadolol**<br>*Corgard* tablet (℞) | Nausea, vomiting, depression, anxiety, chest pain, shortness of breath, swelling, flushing, aching, eye problems, dry mouth. | | May be taken without regard to meals. | May also be used to treat irregular heartbeats, angina, stage fright, and to prevent migraines. |
| **Penbutolol Sulfate**<br>*Levatol* tablet (℞) | Nausea, vomiting, depression, anxiety, chest pain, shortness of breath, swelling, flushing, aching, eye problems, dry mouth. | | May be taken without regard to meals. | |
| **Pindolol**<br>*Visken* tablet (℞) | Nausea, vomiting, depression, anxiety, chest pain, shortness of breath, swelling, flushing, aching, eye problems, dry mouth. | | May be taken without regard to meals. | May also be used to treat irregular heartbeats. |

**ACTION** Beta blockers slow the heart rate, reduce output of the heart at rest and during exercise, and slow conduction of nerve impulses in the heart and other organs. This generally reduces both the resting and exercising heart rates and will lower both resting and exercising blood pressures. These drugs may increase exercise capacity in patients with angina. These products may mask signs of low blood sugar in diabetics. Inform the doctor or dentist of use before any type of surgery.

**INDICATION** Used to lower high blood pressure either alone or in combination with other blood pressure medications.

**BANNED SUBSTANCES** NCAA and/or USOC may list some of these substances as banned for athletes to use.

| Generic Name<br>*Brand Name* | Side Effects | Warnings | Dosing | Notes |
|---|---|---|---|---|
| **Propranolol HCl**<br>*Inderal* tablet (℞)<br>*Inderal LA*<br>  sustained-release<br>  capsule (℞) | Nausea, vomiting, depression, anxiety, chest pain, shortness of breath, swelling, flushing, aching, eye problems, dry mouth. | | Take consistently with or without food at the same time each day. | May also be used to treat irregular heartbeats, heart attacks, tremors, alcohol withdrawal syndrome, stage fright, schizophrenia, anxiety, and to prevent migraines. |
| **Sotalol HCl**<br>*Betapace* tablet (℞) | Nausea, vomiting, depression, anxiety, chest pain, shortness of breath, swelling, flushing, aching, eye problems, dry mouth. | | Take on an empty stomach as food may reduce absorption. | May also be used to treat irregular heartbeats. |
| **Timolol Maleate**<br>*Blocadren* tablet<br>  (℞) | Nausea, vomiting, depression, anxiety, chest pain, shortness of breath, swelling, flushing, aching, eye problems, dry mouth. | | | May also be used to treat irregular heartbeats, tremors, and to prevent migraines. |

# Blood-Modifying Agents

**ACTION** These products affect the ability of blood to clot or flow in the body.

**INDICATION** Used to treat problems associated with blood flow.

| Generic Name<br>*Brand Name* | Side Effects | Warnings | Dosing | Notes |
|---|---|---|---|---|
| **Anagrelide HCl**<br>*Agrylin* capsule (℞) | Headache, diarrhea, GI discomfort, palpitations, edema, nausea, dizziness, dyspepsia, flatulence. | | May take without regard to food. | Used for the treatment of elevated platelet counts in essential thrombocythemia. |
| **Dipyridamole**<br>*Persantine* tablet (℞) | Stomach ache, diarrhea, nausea, dizziness, fainting, flushing. | | May take without regard to food. | Used to prevent blood clots by preventing platelets from clumping. Also used with aspirin to prevent heart attacks. |
| **Pentoxifylline**<br>*Trental* tablet (℞) | Stomachache, constipation, nausea, dizziness, headache, confusion, low blood pressure. | May cause dizziness. Use caution when performing tasks that require alertness. Do not crush or chew tablet. | Take with meals. | Used to improve blood flow in arms and legs by reducing thickness of blood. |
| **Ticlopidine HCl**<br>*Ticlid* tablet (℞) | Diarrhea, nausea, indigestion, bruising, vomiting. | | Take with food to minimize stomach upset. | Used to prevent blood clots by preventing platelets from clumping, reducing the risk of stroke. |
| **Warfarin Sodium**<br>*Coumadin*, *Panwarfin* tablet (℞) | Bleeding, bruising, dark urine, nausea, cramps. | Avoid alcohol, aspirin, and drastic changes in diet. Do not change from one brand to another. | Strict adherence to dosage schedule is important. | Used to prevent blood clot recurrence in the veins. |

Cardiovascular

# Calcium Channel Blocking Agents

**ACTION** Calcium channel blockers interfere with the normal role of calcium in the heart and in blood vessel muscle contraction. They dilate arteries, may decrease or increase heart rate, decrease heart contraction, and slow the ability of the heart to contract. This lowers both resting and exercising blood pressures. These drugs may increase exercise capacity in patients with angina. Calcium channel blockers may cause inhibition of platelet function. Report episodes of bruising to a doctor.

**INDICATION** Used to treat various types of angina and to treat high blood pressure.

| Generic Name<br>*Brand Name* | Side Effects | Warnings | Dosing | Notes |
|---|---|---|---|---|
| **Amlodipine Besylate**<br>*Norvasc* tablet (℞) | Nausea, abdominal cramps, dizziness, headache, weakness, fatigue, edema, flushing, shortness of breath. | | May be taken with or without food. | |
| **Bepridil HCl**<br>*Vascor* tablet (℞) | Nausea, diarrhea, dry mouth, abdominal cramps, dizziness, headache, weakness, anxiety, depression, edema, sweating, shortness of breath. | | May take with meals or at bedtime if stomach upset occurs. | |
| **Diltiazem HCl**<br>*Cardizem* tablet (℞)<br>*Cardizem CD, Dilacor XR, Cardizem SR, Tiazac* sustained-release capsule (℞) | Nausea, abdominal cramps, dizziness, headache, weakness, edema, flushing, shortness of breath, muscle cramps. | Do not crush or chew. | Take sustained-release dose on an empty stomach in the morning. | May be used to treat unstable angina, tardive dyskinesia, and to prevent heart attacks. |
| **Felodipine**<br>*Plendil* sustained-release tablet (℞) | Nausea, abdominal cramps, dizziness, headache, weakness, edema, flushing, shortness of breath. | Do not take with grapefruit juice. | May be taken with or without food. | |

**ACTION** Calcium channel blockers interfere with the normal role of calcium in the heart and in blood vessel muscle contraction. They dilate arteries, may decrease or increase heart rate, decrease heart contraction, and slow the ability of the heart to contract. This lowers both resting and exercising blood pressures. These drugs may increase exercise capacity in patients with angina. Calcium channel blockers may cause inhibition of platelet function. Report episodes of bruising to a doctor.

**INDICATION** Used to treat various types of angina and to treat high blood pressure.

| Generic Name<br>*Brand Name* | Side Effects | Warnings | Dosing | Notes |
|---|---|---|---|---|
| **Isradipine**<br>*DynaCirc* capsule (℞)<br>*DynaCirc CR* controlled-release tablet (℞) | Nausea, abdominal cramps, dizziness, headache, weakness, fatigue, edema, flushing, shortness of breath. | Do not crush or chew tablet. | May be taken with or without food. | May be used in the treatment of chronic stable angina. |
| **Mibefradil HCL**<br>*Posicor* tablet (℞) | Dizziness, headache, leg edema, rhinitis, abdominal pain, dyspepsia, fatigue. | Do not crush or chew tablet. | May be taken with or without food. | |
| **Nifedipine**<br>*Adalat, Procardia* capsule (℞)<br>*Adalat CC, Procardia XL* sustained-release tablet (℞) | Nausea, abdominal cramps, dizziness, headache, weakness, fatigue, edema, flushing, shortness of breath. | It is all right if an empty tablet appears in the stool. | May be taken with or without food. Sustained-release tablet should be taken in morning on an empty stomach. | May be used to prevent migraine headaches and to treat certain types of heart disorders. |
| **Nicardipine HCL**<br>*Cardene* capsule (℞)<br>*Cardene SR* sustained-release capsule (℞) | Nausea, abdominal cramps, dizziness, headache, weakness, drowsiness, edema, flushing. | | May be taken with or without food. | May be useful in the treatment of congestive heart failure. |
| **Nimodipine**<br>*Nimotop* liquid, capsule (℞) | Nausea, abdominal cramps, headache, edema, flushing, shortness of breath. | | Do not take within 1 hour before or 2 hours after meals. | May be used to improve neurological deficiencies caused by ruptured vessels in the brain. May be useful for chronic cluster headaches. |

**ACTION** Calcium channel blockers interfere with the normal role of calcium in the heart and in blood vessel muscle contraction. They dilate arteries, may decrease or increase heart rate, decrease heart contraction, and slow the ability of the heart to contract. This lowers both resting and exercising blood pressures. These drugs may increase exercise capacity in patients with angina. Calcium channel blockers may cause inhibition of platelet function. Report episodes of bruising to a doctor.

**INDICATION** Used to treat various types of angina and to treat high blood pressure.

| Generic Name<br>*Brand Name* | Side Effects | Warnings | Dosing | Notes |
|---|---|---|---|---|
| **Nisoldipine**<br>*Sular* sustained-<br>release tablet (℞) | Nausea, ab-<br>dominal cramps,<br>dizziness, head-<br>ache, weakness,<br>fatigue, edema,<br>flushing, short-<br>ness of breath,<br>acne, pharyngitis. | Do not crush or<br>chew tablet. Do<br>not take with<br>grapefruit juice<br>or high fat meals. | | |
| **Verapamil HCL**<br>*Calan, Isoptin*<br>tablet (℞)<br>*Calan SR,*<br>*Isoptin SR,*<br>*Covera-HS*<br>sustained-release<br>tablet (℞)<br>*Verelan* sustained-<br>release capsule<br>(℞) | Nausea, ab-<br>dominal cramps,<br>dizziness, head-<br>ache, weakness,<br>fatigue, edema,<br>flushing, short-<br>ness of breath. | It is all right if an<br>empty tablet<br>appears in<br>the stool. | May be taken<br>with or without<br>food. | May be used to<br>prevent migraine<br>headaches,<br>cluster head-<br>aches, exercise-<br>induced asthma,<br>and to treat leg<br>cramps and<br>manic-<br>depressive<br>states. |

## Cardiac Glycosides

**ACTION** Cardiac glycosides increase the heart's output and the force with which the heart pumps and improves the blood circulation. They also reduce swelling and fluid retention due to congestive heart failure, as well as slow and steady the heart rate. Cardiac glycosides may decrease the heart rate and increase exercise capacity in patients with congestive heart failure. Do not switch from one brand to another; products manufactured by different companies may not be equally effective.

**INDICATION** Used to treat congestive heart failure and certain heart conditions where the heart is beating too fast or too irregularly to function.

| Generic Name<br>*Brand Name* | Side Effects | Warnings | Dosing | Notes |
|---|---|---|---|---|
| **Digitoxin**<br>*Crystodigin*<br>tablet (R) | Loss of appetite, weakness, headache, depression, visual disturbances, drowsiness, confusion. | Avoid antacids, cough, cold, allergy, and diet drugs, except on professional advice. | | |
| **Digoxin**<br>*Lanoxin* tablet (R)<br>*Lanoxicaps*<br>capsule (R) | Loss of appetite, weakness, headache, depression, visual disturbances, drowsiness, confusion. | Avoid antacids, cough, cold, allergy, and diet drugs, except on professional advice. | | |

Cardiovascular

## Diuretics

**ACTION** Diuretics cause electrolytes and water to be excreted by the kidneys. Potassium supplements may be necessary with some diuretics, while others reduce the amount of potassium excreted. Although lowering fluid volume in the body may have no effect on heart rate, it may reduce both resting and exercising blood pressures. Diuretics may increase exercise capacity in patients with congestive heart failure.

**INDICATION** Used to treat edema due to congestive heart failure, liver disease, or kidney disease.

**BANNED SUBSTANCES** NCAA and/or USOC may list some of these substances as banned for athletes to use.

| Generic Name<br>*Brand Name* | Side Effects | Warnings | Dosing | Notes |
|---|---|---|---|---|
| **Acetazolamide**<br>*Diamox, AK-Zol*<br>tablet (℞)<br>*Diamox* sustained-<br>release capsule<br>(℞) | Loss of appetite, nausea, vomiting, weakness, fever, weight loss. | May cause drowsiness. | If stomach upset occurs, take with food. | Used to treat glaucoma by reducing fluid formation in the inner eye. |
| **Amiloride HCI**<br>*Midamor* tablet (℞) | Stomach cramps, black, tarlike stools, nausea, weakness, fatigue, chest pain, shortness of breath, deepening of the voice. | Avoid large quantities of potassium-rich food. May cause dizziness or visual disturbances. | If stomach upset occurs, take with food. | Used to treat high blood pressure and to prevent low potassium levels due to other medications. |
| **Bendroflume-**<br>**thiazide**<br>*Naturetin* tablet (℞) | Weakness, cramps, dry mouth, diarrhea, constipation, nausea, orthostatic hypotension, sensitivity to sun, reduced sexual drive, joint pain, fever. | Increases urination so take early in the day. May increase blood sugar levels in diabetics and cause gout attacks. May cause loss of potassium. | If stomach upset occurs, take with food or milk. | Used to treat high blood pressure. |

**ACTION** Diuretics cause electrolytes and water to be excreted by the kidneys. Potassium supplements may be necessary with some diuretics, while others reduce the amount of potassium excreted. Although lowering fluid volume in the body may have no effect on heart rate, it may reduce both resting and exercising blood pressures. Diuretics may increase exercise capacity in patients with congestive heart failure.

**INDICATION** Used to treat edema due to congestive heart failure, liver disease, or kidney disease.

**BANNED SUBSTANCES** NCAA and/or USOC may list some of these substances as banned for athletes to use.

| Generic Name<br>*Brand Name* | Side Effects | Warnings | Dosing | Notes |
|---|---|---|---|---|
| **Benzthiazide**<br>*Aquatag, Proaqua,*<br>*Hydrex, Marazide*<br>tablet (℞) | Weakness, cramps, dry mouth, diarrhea, constipation, nausea, orthostatic hypotension, sensitivity to sun, reduced sexual drive, joint pain, fever. | Increases urination so take early in the day. May increase blood sugar levels in diabetics and cause gout attacks. May cause loss of potassium. | If stomach upset occurs, take with food or milk. | Used to treat high blood pressure. |
| **Bumetanide**<br>*Bumex* tablet (℞) | Weakness, dizziness, loss of appetite, diarrhea, nausea, vomiting, restlessness, weak pulse, sweating, dehydration, joint pain, fever, blurred vision. | May make you sensitive to the sun. May increase blood glucose levels in diabetics. Drug will increase urination so take early in the day. | If stomach upset occurs, take with food or milk. | |
| **Chlorothiazide**<br>*Diuril* tablet (℞) | Weakness, cramps, dry mouth, diarrhea, constipation, nausea, orthostatic hypotension, sensitivity to sun, reduced sexual drive, joint pain, fever. | Increases urination so take early in the day. May increase blood sugar levels in diabetics and cause gout attacks. May cause loss of potassium. | If stomach upset occurs, take with food or milk. | Used to treat high blood pressure. |

**ACTION** Diuretics cause electrolytes and water to be excreted by the kidneys. Potassium supplements may be necessary with some diuretics, while others reduce the amount of potassium excreted. Although lowering fluid volume in the body may have no effect on heart rate, it may reduce both resting and exercising blood pressures. Diuretics may increase exercise capacity in patients with congestive heart failure.

**INDICATION** Used to treat edema due to congestive heart failure, liver disease, or kidney disease.

**BANNED SUBSTANCES** NCAA and/or USOC may list some of these substances as banned for athletes to use.

| Generic Name<br>*Brand Name* | Side Effects | Warnings | Dosing | Notes |
|---|---|---|---|---|
| **Chlorthalidone**<br>*Hygroton* tablet (℞) | Weakness, cramps, dry mouth, diarrhea, constipation, nausea, orthostatic hypotension, sensitivity to sun, reduced sexual drive, joint pain, fever. | Increases urination so take early in the day. May increase blood sugar levels in diabetics and cause gout attacks. May cause loss of potassium. | If stomach upset occurs, take with food or milk. | Used to treat high blood pressure. |
| **Dichlorphena-mide**<br>*Daranide* tablet (℞) | Loss of appetite, nausea, vomiting, weakness, fever, weight loss. | May cause drowsiness. | If stomach upset occurs, take with food. | Used to treat glaucoma by reducing fluid formation in the inner eye. |
| **Ethacrynic Acid**<br>*Edecrin* tablet (℞) | Weakness, dizziness, loss of appetite, diarrhea, nausea, vomiting, restlessness, weak pulse, sweating, dehydration, joint pain, fever, blurred vision. | Drug will increase urination so take early in the day. May increase sensitivity to the sun. May increase blood glucose levels in diabetics. | If stomach upset occurs, take with food or milk. | Used to treat fluid accumulation due to cancer and other conditions. |

**ACTION** Diuretics cause electrolytes and water to be excreted by the kidneys. Potassium supplements may be necessary with some diuretics, while others reduce the amount of potassium excreted. Although lowering fluid volume in the body may have no effect on heart rate, it may reduce both resting and exercising blood pressures. Diuretics may increase exercise capacity in patients with congestive heart failure.

**INDICATION** Used to treat edema due to congestive heart failure, liver disease, or kidney disease.

**BANNED SUBSTANCES** NCAA and/or USOC may list some of these substances as banned for athletes to use.

| Generic Name<br>*Brand Name* | Side Effects | Warnings | Dosing | Notes |
|---|---|---|---|---|
| **Furosemide**<br>*Lasix* tablet,<br> solution (℞) | Weakness, dizziness, loss of appetite, diarrhea, nausea, vomiting, restlessness, weak pulse, sweating, dehydration, joint pain, fever, blurred vision. | Drug will increase urination so take early in the day. May increase sensitivity to the sun. May increase blood glucose levels in diabetics. | If stomach upset occurs, take with food or milk. | Used to treat hypertension and fluid accumulation in the lungs. |
| **Hydrochlorothiazide**<br>*HCTZ, Esidrix,*<br>*Hydrodiuril, Oretic*<br> tablet (℞) | Weakness, cramps, dry mouth, diarrhea, constipation, nausea, orthostatic hypotension, sensitivity to sun, reduced sexual drive, joint pain, fever. | Increases urination so take early in the day. May increase blood sugar levels in diabetics and cause gout attacks. May cause loss of potassium. | If stomach upset occurs, take with food or milk. | Used to treat high blood pressure. |
| **Hydroflumethiazide**<br>*Diucardin, Saluron*<br> tablet (℞) | Weakness, cramps, dry mouth, diarrhea, constipation, nausea, orthostatic hypotension, sensitivity to sun, reduced sexual drive, joint pain, fever. | Increases urination so take early in the day. May increase blood sugar levels in diabetics and cause gout attacks. May cause loss of potassium. | If stomach upset occurs, take with food or milk. | Used to treat high blood pressure. |

Cardiovascular

**ACTION** Diuretics cause electrolytes and water to be excreted by the kidneys. Potassium supplements may be necessary with some diuretics, while others reduce the amount of potassium excreted. Although lowering fluid volume in the body may have no effect on heart rate, it may reduce both resting and exercising blood pressures. Diuretics may increase exercise capacity in patients with congestive heart failure.

**INDICATION** Used to treat edema due to congestive heart failure, liver disease, or kidney disease.

**BANNED SUBSTANCES** NCAA and/or USOC may list some of these substances as banned for athletes to use.

| Generic Name<br>*Brand Name* | Side Effects | Warnings | Dosing | Notes |
|---|---|---|---|---|
| **Indapamide**<br>*Lozol* tablet (℞) | Weakness, cramps, dry mouth, diarrhea, constipation, nausea, orthostatic hypotension, sensitivity to sun, reduced sexual drive, joint pain, fever. | Increases urination so take early in the day. May increase blood sugar levels in diabetics and cause gout attacks. May cause loss of potassium. | If stomach upset occurs, take with food or milk. | Used to treat high blood pressure. |
| **Methazolamide**<br>*Neptazane*<br>tablet (℞) | Loss of appetite, nausea, vomiting, weakness, fever, weight loss. | May cause drowsiness. | If stomach upset occurs, take with food. | Used to treat glaucoma by reducing fluid formation in the inner eye. |
| **Methyclothiazide**<br>*Aquatensen,*<br>*Enduron* tablet (℞) | Weakness, cramps, dry mouth, diarrhea, constipation, nausea, orthostatic hypotension, sensitivity to sun, reduced sexual drive, joint pain, fever. | Increases urination so take early in the day. May increase blood sugar levels in diabetics and cause gout attacks. May cause loss of potassium. | If stomach upset occurs, take with food or milk. | Used to treat high blood pressure. |

**ACTION** Diuretics cause electrolytes and water to be excreted by the kidneys. Potassium supplements may be necessary with some diuretics, while others reduce the amount of potassium excreted. Although lowering fluid volume in the body may have no effect on heart rate, it may reduce both resting and exercising blood pressures. Diuretics may increase exercise capacity in patients with congestive heart failure.

**INDICATION** Used to treat edema due to congestive heart failure, liver disease, or kidney disease.

**BANNED SUBSTANCES** NCAA and/or USOC may list some of these substances as banned for athletes to use.

| Generic Name<br>*Brand Name* | Side Effects | Warnings | Dosing | Notes |
|---|---|---|---|---|
| **Metolazone**<br>*Mykrox, Zaroxolyn*<br>tablet (℞) | Weakness, cramps, dry mouth, diarrhea, constipation, nausea, orthostatic hypotension, sensitivity to sun, reduced sexual drive, joint pain, fever. | Increases urination so take early in the day. May increase blood sugar levels in diabetics and cause gout attacks. May cause loss of potassium. | If stomach upset occurs, take with food or milk. | Used to treat high blood pressure. |
| **Polythiazide**<br>*Renese* tablet (℞) | Weakness, cramps, dry mouth, diarrhea, constipation, nausea, orthostatic hypotension, sensitivity to sun, reduced sexual drive, joint pain, fever. | Increases urination so take early in the day. May increase blood sugar levels in diabetics and cause gout attacks. May cause loss of potassium. | If stomach upset occurs, take with food or milk. | Used to treat high blood pressure. |
| **Quinethazone**<br>*Hydromox* tablet (℞) | Weakness, cramps, dry mouth, diarrhea, constipation, nausea, orthostatic hypotension, sensitivity to sun, reduced sexual drive, joint pain, fever. | Increases urination so take early in the day. May increase blood sugar levels in diabetics and cause gout attacks. May cause loss of potassium. | If stomach upset occurs, take with food or milk. | Used to treat high blood pressure. |

Cardiovascular

**ACTION** Diuretics cause electrolytes and water to be excreted by the kidneys. Potassium supplements may be necessary with some diuretics, while others reduce the amount of potassium excreted. Although lowering fluid volume in the body may have no effect on heart rate, it may reduce both resting and exercising blood pressures. Diuretics may increase exercise capacity in patients with congestive heart failure.

**INDICATION** Used to treat edema due to congestive heart failure, liver disease, or kidney disease.

**BANNED SUBSTANCES** NCAA and/or USOC may list some of these substances as banned for athletes to use.

| Generic Name<br>*Brand Name* | Side Effects | Warnings | Dosing | Notes |
|---|---|---|---|---|
| **Spironolactone**<br>*Aldactone* tablet<br>(℞) | Stomach cramps, black, tarlike stools, nausea, weakness, fatigue, chest pain, shortness of breath, deepening of the voice. | May cause drowsiness and mental confusion. | | Used to treat high blood pressure and to prevent low potassium levels due to other medications and to treat primary hyperaldosteronism. |
| **Torsemide**<br>*Dermadex* tablet (℞) | Weakness, dizziness, loss of appetite, diarrhea, nausea, vomiting, restlessness, weak pulse, sweating, dehydration, joint pain, fever, blurred vision. | Drug will increase urination so take early in the day. May increase sensitivity to the sun. May increase blood glucose levels in diabetics. | May take regardless of meals. | Used to treat hypertension and fluid accumulation in the lungs. |
| **Triamterene**<br>*Dyrenium* capsule (℞) | Stomach cramps, black, tarlike stools, nausea, weakness, fatigue, chest pain, shortness of breath, deepening of the voice. | Avoid prolonged exposure to sunlight. | If upsets stomach, take after meals. If taking a single daily dose, take in the morning. | Used to treat high blood pressure and to prevent low potassium levels due to other medications. |

**ACTION** Diuretics cause electrolytes and water to be excreted by the kidneys. Potassium supplements may be necessary with some diuretics, while others reduce the amount of potassium excreted. Although lowering fluid volume in the body may have no effect on heart rate, it may reduce both resting and exercising blood pressures. Diuretics may increase exercise capacity in patients with congestive heart failure.

**INDICATION** Used to treat edema due to congestive heart failure, liver disease, or kidney disease.

**BANNED SUBSTANCES** NCAA and/or USOC may list some of these substances as banned for athletes to use.

| Generic Name<br>*Brand Name* | Side Effects | Warnings | Dosing | Notes |
|---|---|---|---|---|
| **Trichlormethia-zide**<br>*Diurese, Naqua*<br>tablet (℞) | Weakness, cramps, dry mouth, diarrhea, constipation, nausea, orthostatic hypotension, sensitivity to sun, reduced sexual drive, joint pain, fever. | Increases urination so take early in the day. May increase blood sugar levels in diabetics and cause gout attacks. May cause loss of potassium. | If stomach upset occurs, take with food or milk. | Used to treat high blood pressure. |

## Peripheral Vasodilators

**ACTION** Peripheral vasodilators improve blood flow and supply by causing blood vessels to dilate or widen. Peripheral vasodilators may have no effect on heart rate, but may decrease blood pressure, with little effect on exercise capacity.

**INDICATION** Used to treat disorders related to inadequate blood supply to the arms and legs.

| Generic Name<br>*Brand Name* | Side Effects | Warnings | Dosing | Notes |
|---|---|---|---|---|
| **Cyclandelate**<br>*Cyclan,*<br>*Cyclospasmol*<br>tablet, capsule<br>(℞) | Chest pain, weakness, flushing, headache, belching, heartburn. | | Take with food or antacids if heartburn or stomach upset occurs. | May be used for leg cramps, vertigo, migraines, dementia, and diabetic peripheral polyneuropathy. |

Cardiovascular

**ACTION** Peripheral vasodilators improve blood flow and supply by causing blood vessels to dilate or widen. Peripheral vasodilators may have no effect on heart rate, but may decrease blood pressure, with little effect on exercise capacity.

**INDICATION** Used to treat disorders related to inadequate blood supply to the arms and legs.

| Generic Name<br>Brand Name | Side Effects | Warnings | Dosing | Notes |
|---|---|---|---|---|
| **Isoxsuprine HCl**<br>*Vasodilan*<br>tablet (℞) | Orthostatic hypotension, chest pain, severe rash, flushing, dizziness, weakness, nausea. | Notify a doctor if flushing, skin rash, or a pounding sensation in chest occurs. | | May be used for painful menstrual periods and premature labor. |
| **Nylidrin HCl**<br>*Arlidin* tablet (℞) | Nervousness, weakness, dizziness, nausea, vomiting. | May cause drowsiness. | | May be used for leg cramps, frostbite, and circulatory problems in the ear. |
| **Papaverine HCL**<br>*Pavabid, Cerespan*<br>timed-release capsule (℞) | Nausea, appetite loss, headache, flushing, fatigue. | May cause drowsiness. | Take at evenly spaced intervals throughout the day. | |

## Antihypertensive Agents— Miscellaneous

**ACTION** These products work primarily by relaxing and dilating blood vessels, which allows the blood to flow more freely at a lower pressure. This generally has no effect on the heart rate, but does lower both resting and exercising blood pressures.

**INDICATION** Used to lower high blood pressure either alone or in combination with other blood pressure medications.

| Generic Name<br>Brand Name | Side Effects | Warnings | Dosing | Notes |
|---|---|---|---|---|
| **Carvedilol**<br>*Coreg* tablet (℞) | Stomach pain, diarrhea, dizziness, slow heart rate, runny nose, sore throat, fatigue. | Contact lens wearers may experience reduced lacrimation. | Take with food to slow rate of absorption and to reduce lightheadedness. | May also be used for congestive heart failure and chest pain. |

**ACTION** These products work primarily by relaxing and dilating blood vessels, which allows the blood to flow more freely at a lower pressure. This generally has no effect on the heart rate, but does lower both resting and exercising blood pressures.

**INDICATION** Used to lower high blood pressure either alone or in combination with other blood pressure medications.

| Generic Name Brand Name | Side Effects | Warnings | Dosing | Notes |
|---|---|---|---|---|
| **Clonidine** *Catapres* tablet (℞) *Catapres TTS* transdermal patch (℞) | Constipation, nausea, depression, orthostatic hypotension, hair thinning, dry mouth, loss of sex drive. | Alcohol may cause excessive drowsiness. Do not stop taking this drug suddenly. Dose must be reduced gradually. | | May also be used for alcohol withdrawal, diabetic diarrhea, ulcerative colitis, menopausal flushing, and Tourette's syndrome. |
| **Guanabenz Acetate** *Wytensin* tablet (℞) | Nausea, vomiting, depression, dizziness, chest pain, shortness of breath, edema, blurred vision. | Use of alcohol may cause excessive drowsiness. | | Avoid cough, cold, or allergy medications except on professional recommendation. |
| **Guanadrel Sulfate** *Hylorel* tablet (℞) | Severe diarrhea, indigestion, headache, chest pain, cough, ankle swelling, leg cramps, dry mouth. | Dizziness is common. Excess heat can worsen the dizziness. | | |
| **Guanethidine Monosulfate** *Ismelin* tablet (℞) | Dizziness, weakness, diarrhea, chest pain, hair loss, blurred vision. | Dizziness is common. Excess heat can worsen the dizziness. | | May also be used for high blood pressure caused by certain kidney diseases. |
| **Guanfacine HCL** *Tenex* tablet (℞) | Constipation, nausea, memory loss, confusion, slow pulse, shortness of breath, drowsiness, sweating. | Alcohol may intensify drowsiness. | Take at bedtime to reduce daytime sedation. | |

Cardiovascular

**ACTION** These products work primarily by relaxing and dilating blood vessels, which allows the blood to flow more freely at a lower pressure. This generally has no effect on the heart rate, but does lower both resting and exercising blood pressures.

**INDICATION** Used to lower high blood pressure either alone or in combination with other blood pressure medications.

| Generic Name<br>*Brand Name* | Side Effects | Warnings | Dosing | Notes |
|---|---|---|---|---|
| **Hydralazine**<br>*Apresoline* tablet<br>(℞) | Nausea, vomiting, headache, chest pain, flushing, joint pain, muscle aches. | | Take with meals. | May also be used for congestive heart failure and after valve replacement. |
| **Labetalol HCL**<br>*Normodyne,*<br>*Trandate* tablet (℞) | Nausea, vomiting, dizziness, fatigue, hair loss, difficult breathing, wheezing, muscle cramps. | Do not abruptly stop this medication. | May be taken with or without food, but should be taken the same way each time. | May also be used for pheochromocytoma and clonidine withdrawal. |
| **Losartan Potassium**<br>*Cozaar* tablet (℞) | Diarrhea, indigestion, nausea, cough, stuffy nose, dizziness, sleeplessness, fluid retention. | Dehydration may increase the blood-lowering effect causing dizziness. | May be taken without regard to food. | |
| **Mecamylamine**<br>*Inversine* tablet (℞) | Nausea, vomiting, convulsions, weakness, fatigue, decreased sexual function, dry mouth, blurred vision. | Do not restrict dietary salt. | Take after meals. | |
| **Methyldopa**<br>*Aldomet* tablet (℞) | Nausea, vomiting, dizziness, chest pain, shortness of breath, edema, decreased sex drive, anemia. | Use of alcohol may cause excessive drowsiness. | | |

**ACTION** These products work primarily by relaxing and dilating blood vessels, which allows the blood to flow more freely at a lower pressure. This generally has no effect on the heart rate, but does lower both resting and exercising blood pressures.

**INDICATION** Used to lower high blood pressure either alone or in combination with other blood pressure medications.

| Generic Name<br>*Brand Name* | Side Effects | Warnings | Dosing | Notes |
|---|---|---|---|---|
| **Minoxidil**<br>*Loniten* tablet (℞) | Nausea, vomiting, dizziness, headache, chest pain, shortness of breath, increased hair growth, weight gain, swelling. | Notify a doctor if increased heart rate, unusual swelling, breathing difficulty, new chest pain, or fainting occurs. | A low-salt diet should be closely followed. | Used topically for promoting hair growth. |
| **Reserpine**<br>*Serpasil* tablet (℞) | Nausea, vomiting, drowsiness, dizziness, blurred vision, depression, chest pain, shortness of breath, changes in sex drive, eye problems. | Avoid tyramine-containing foods (e.g., cheddar cheese, yogurt, raisins). | Take with food; may cause stomach upset. | Used to relieve symptoms in agitated mental states. |
| **Valsartan**<br>*Diovan* (℞) | Insomnia, dyspepsia, impotence, vertigo, palpitations, abdominal pain. | | Take with or without food. | |

Cardiovascular

## Combination Cardiovascular Medications

Many cardiovascular medications are combined with a second medication. Most combinations include a diuretic. The nondiuretic portion can be any of the cardiovascular medications in this chapter.

**BANNED SUBSTANCES** NCAA and/or USOC may list some of these substances as banned for athletes to use.

| Brand Name | Nondiuretic | Diuretic |
|---|---|---|
| Aldactazide (R) | None | Spironolactone, Hydrochlorothiazide |
| Aldoclor (R) | Methyldopa | Chlorothiazide |
| Aldoril (R) | Methyldopa | Hydrochlorothiazide |
| Aldoril-D (R) | Methyldopa | Hydrochlorothiazide |
| Apresazide (R) | Hydralazine | Hydrochlorothiazide |
| Capozide (R) | Captopril | Hydrochlorothiazide |
| Combipres (R) | Clonidine | Chlorthalidone |
| Corzide (R) | Nadolol | Bendroflumethiazide |
| Demi-Regroton (R) | Reserpine | Chlorthalidone |
| Diupres (R) | Reserpine | Chlorothiazide |
| Diutensen-R (R) | Reserpine | Methyclothiazide |
| Dyazide (R) | None | Triamterene, Hydrochlorothiazide |
| Enduronyl (R) | Deserpidine | Methyclothiazide |
| Enduronyl Forte (R) | Deserpidine | Methyclothiazide |
| Esimil (R) | Guanethidine Monosulfate | Hydrochlorothiazide |
| Hydropres (R) | Reserpine | Hydrochlorothiazide |
| Hydroserpine (R) | Reserpine | Hydrochlorothiazide |
| Hyzaar (R) | Losartan Potassium | Hydrochlorothiazide |
| Inderide (R) | Propranolol | Hydrochlorothiazide |
| Inderide LA (R) | Propranolol | Hydrochlorothiazide |
| Lexxel (R) | Enalapril Maleate, Felodipine | None |

Many cardiovascular medications are combined with a second medication. Most combinations include a diuretic. The nondiuretic portion can be any of the cardiovascular medications in this chapter.

**BANNED SUBSTANCES** NCAA and/or USOC may list some of these substances as banned for athletes to use.

| Brand Name | Nondiuretic | Diuretic |
|---|---|---|
| Lopressor HCT (℞) | **Metoprolol Tartrate** | **Hydrochlorothiazide** |
| Lotensin HCT (℞) | **Benazepril** | **Hydrochlorothiazide** |
| Lotrel (℞) | **Amlodipine, Benazepril** | None |
| Maxzide (℞) | None | **Triamterene, Hydrochlorothiazide** |
| Metatensin (℞) | **Reserpine** | **Trichlormethiazide** |
| Minizide (℞) | **Prazosin** | **Polythiazide** |
| Moduretic (℞) | None | **Amiloride, Hydrochlorothiazide** |
| Prinzide (℞) | **Lisinopril** | **Hydrochlorothiazide** |
| Rauzide (℞) | **Rauwolfia Serpentina** | **Bendroflumethiazide** |
| Regroton (℞) | **Reserpine** | **Chlorthalidone** |
| Renese-R (℞) | **Reserpine** | **Polythiazide** |
| Salutensin (℞) | **Reserpine** | **Hydroflumethiazide** |
| Ser-Ap-Es (℞) | **Hydralazine, Reserpine** | **Hydrochlorothiazide** |
| Spirozide (℞) | None | **Spironolactone, Hydrochlorothiazide** |
| Teczem (℞) | **Diltiazem, Enalapril Maleate** | None |
| Tenoretic (℞) | **Atenolol** | **Chlorthalidone** |
| Timolide (℞) | **Timolol Maleate** | **Hydrochlorothiazide** |
| Vaseretic (℞) | **Enalapril** | **Hydrochlorothiazide** |
| Zestoretic (℞) | **Lisinopril** | **Hydrochlorothiazide** |
| Ziac (℞) | **Bisoprolol Fumarate** | **Hydrochlorothiazide** |

Cardiovascular

# Gastrointestinal and Urinary Agents

## Antacids

**ACTION** Reduce or neutralize stomach acids and prevent stomach acids from getting into the esophagus thereby reducing heartburn and indigestion. Antacids reduce acidity for about 30 minutes when taken on an empty stomach and for about 3 hours when taken 1 hour after a meal.

**INDICATION** Used for heartburn, acid indigestion, sour stomach, peptic ulcer, and hiatal hernia. Care must be exercised to avoid taking antacids within 1 to 2 hours of other medications as antacids may block the absorption of many other medications.

| Generic Name<br>*Brand Name* | Side Effects | Warnings | Dosing | Notes |
|---|---|---|---|---|
| **Aluminum Carbonate** *Basaljel* capsule, tablet, suspension (OTC) | Nausea, vomiting, constipation, appetite loss, lack of energy. | Notify a doctor if black, tarlike stools or "coffee-ground" vomiting occurs. | Do not take for longer than 2 weeks for indigestion. | May be used to reduce phosphorus levels in certain kidney diseases. |
| **Aluminum Hydroxide** *Amphojel, Alternagel, Alu-Cap* capsule, tablet, suspension (OTC) | Nausea, vomiting, constipation, appetite loss, lack of energy. | Notify a doctor if black, tarlike stools or "coffee-ground" vomiting occurs. | Do not take for longer than 2 weeks for indigestion. | May be used to reduce phosphorus levels in certain kidney diseases. |
| **Aluminum Hydroxide, Magnesium Hydroxide** *Maalox* tablet, suspension (OTC) | Nausea, vomiting, diarrhea, constipation, appetite loss, lack of energy. | Notify a doctor if black, tarlike stools or "coffee-ground" vomiting occurs. | Do not take for longer than 2 weeks for indigestion. | |
| **Aluminum Hydroxide, Magnesium Hydroxide, Simethicone** *Mylanta, Gelusil, Maalox Plus, Di-Gel* tablet, liquid (OTC) | Nausea, vomiting, diarrhea, constipation, appetite loss, lack of energy. | Notify a doctor if black, tarlike stools or "coffee-ground" vomiting occurs. | Do not take for longer than 2 weeks for indigestion. | Simethicone added to reduce gastrointestinal gas and bloating. |

**ACTION** Reduce or neutralize stomach acids and prevent stomach acids from getting into the esophagus thereby reducing heartburn and indigestion. Antacids reduce acidity for about 30 minutes when taken on an empty stomach and for about 3 hours when taken 1 hour after a meal.

**INDICATION** Used for heartburn, acid indigestion, sour stomach, peptic ulcer, and hiatal hernia. Care must be exercised to avoid taking antacids within 1 to 2 hours of other medications as antacids may block the absorption of many other medications.

| Generic Name<br>*Brand Name* | Side Effects | Warnings | Dosing | Notes |
|---|---|---|---|---|
| **Calcium Carbonate**<br>*Tums, Chooz*<br>tablet (OTC) | Nausea, vomiting, constipation, appetite loss, lack of energy. | Notify a doctor if black, tarlike stools or "coffee-ground" vomiting occurs. | Do not take for longer than 2 weeks for indigestion. | May be used to treat calcium deficiencies. |
| **Dihydroxy-aluminum Sodium Carbonate**<br>*Rolaids* tablet (OTC) | Nausea, vomiting, constipation, appetite loss, lack of energy. | Notify a doctor if black, tarlike stools or "coffee-ground" vomiting occurs. | Do not take for longer than 2 weeks for indigestion. | May be used to reduce phosphorus levels in certain kidney diseases. |
| **Magaldrate**<br>*Riopan* tablet, suspension (OTC) | Nausea, vomiting, constipation, appetite loss, lack of energy. | Notify a doctor if black, tarlike stools or "coffee-ground" vomiting occurs. | Do not take for longer than 2 weeks for indigestion. | |
| **Magnesium Hydroxide**<br>*Milk of Magnesia* tablet, suspension (OTC) | Nausea, vomiting, diarrhea, appetite loss, lack of energy. | Notify a doctor if black, tarlike stools or "coffee-ground" vomiting occurs. | Do not take for longer than 2 weeks for indigestion. | May also be used as a laxative. |
| **Magnesium Oxide**<br>*Mag-Ox* tablet (OTC) | Nausea, vomiting, constipation, appetite loss, lack of energy. | Notify a doctor if black, tarlike stools or "coffee-ground" vomiting occurs. | Do not take for longer than 2 weeks for indigestion. | |
| **Sodium Bicarbonate, Citric Acid, Aspirin**<br>*Alka-Seltzer* (original formulation) effervescent tablet (OTC) | Nausea, vomiting, diarrhea, constipation, appetite loss, lack of energy. | Notify a doctor if black, tarlike stools or "coffee-ground" vomiting occurs. | Allow to completely dissolve in water and for bubbling to stop before drinking. | These are numerous formulations of Alka-Seltzer available. Care should be taken to understand which medications are in the product being used. |

Gastrointestinal & Urinary

# Anticholinergics/Antispasmodics

**ACTION** These drugs typically slow the activity of the stomach and intestine, reduce cramping, reduce secretions, and relax the urinary bladder. They also may slow or increase the heart rate, block sweating, which may increase body temperature, and dilate the pupils of the eyes.

**INDICATION** As a group these medications may be used for peptic ulcers, diarrhea, colic, urinary problems, and motion sickness, as well as other disorders.

| Generic Name<br>*Brand Name* | Side Effects | Warnings | Dosing | Notes |
|---|---|---|---|---|
| **Anisotropine Methylbromide**<br>*Valpin* tablet (℞) | Nausea, vomiting, constipation, confusion, excitement, pulse changes, nasal congestion, flushing, dry mouth. | May cause drowsiness. | Take 30 minutes before meals. | |
| **Atropine Sulfate**<br>*Atropine Sulfate* tablet (℞) | Nausea, vomiting, constipation, confusion, excitement, pulse changes, nasal congestion, flushing, dry mouth. | May cause drowsiness. | Take 30 minutes before meals. | |
| **Atropine Sulfate, Scopolamine, Hyoscyamine, Phenobarbital**<br>*Donnatal, Kinesed, Relaxadon* tablet, elixir (℞) | Nausea, vomiting, constipation, confusion, excitement, pulse changes, nasal congestion, flushing, dry mouth. | May cause drowsiness. | Take 30 minutes before meals. | |
| **Belladonna Alkaloids**<br>*Belladonna* tablet, liquid (℞) | Nausea, vomiting, constipation, confusion, excitement, pulse changes, nasal congestion, flushing, dry mouth. | May cause drowsiness. | Take 30 minutes before meals. | |

**ACTION** These drugs typically slow the activity of the stomach and intestine, reduce cramping, reduce secretions, and relax the urinary bladder. They also may slow or increase the heart rate, block sweating, which may increase body temperature, and dilate the pupils of the eyes.

**INDICATION** As a group these medications may be used for peptic ulcers, diarrhea, colic, urinary problems, and motion sickness, as well as other disorders.

| Generic Name<br>*Brand Name* | Side Effects | Warnings | Dosing | Notes |
|---|---|---|---|---|
| **Belladonna Alkaloids, Phenobarbital**<br>*Bellergal-S, Belladenal* tablet<br>(℞) | Nausea, vomiting, constipation, confusion, excitement, pulse changes, nasal congestion, flushing, dry mouth. | May cause drowsiness. | Take 30 minutes before meals. | |
| **Belladonna Alkaloids, Butabarbital**<br>*Butibel* tablet (℞) | Nausea, vomiting, constipation, confusion, excitement, pulse changes, nasal congestion, flushing, dry mouth. | May cause drowsiness. | Take 30 minutes before meals. | |
| **Clidinium Bromide**<br>*Quarzan* capsule<br>(℞) | Nausea, vomiting, constipation, confusion, excitement, pulse changes, nasal congestion, flushing, dry mouth. | May cause drowsiness. | Take 30 minutes before meals. | |
| **Clidinium Bromide, Chlordiazepoxide**<br>*Librax, Clindex* capsule (℞) | Nausea, vomiting, constipation, confusion, excitement, pulse changes, nasal congestion, flushing, dry mouth. | May cause drowsiness; alcohol and other depressants may intensify this effect. | Take 30 minutes before meals. | |
| **Dicyclomine**<br>*Bentyl* tablet, capsule (℞) | Nausea, vomiting, constipation, confusion, excitement, pulse changes, nasal congestion, flushing, dry mouth. | May cause drowsiness. | Take 30 minutes before meals. | |

Gastrointestinal & Urinary

**ACTION** These drugs typically slow the activity of the stomach and intestine, reduce cramping, reduce secretions, and relax the urinary bladder. They also may slow or increase the heart rate, block sweating, which may increase body temperature, and dilate the pupils of the eyes.

**INDICATION** As a group these medications may be used for peptic ulcers, diarrhea, colic, urinary problems, and motion sickness, as well as other disorders.

| Generic Name<br>Brand Name | Side Effects | Warnings | Dosing | Notes |
|---|---|---|---|---|
| **Glycopyrrolate**<br>*Robinul* tablet (℞) | Nausea, vomiting, constipation, confusion, excitement, pulse changes, nasal congestion, flushing, dry mouth. | May cause drowsiness. | Take 30 minutes before meals. | For treatment of peptic ulcer only. |
| **Hyoscyamine Sulfate**<br>*Anaspaz, Levsin, Cystospaz, Levsinex* tablet, capsules, solution (℞) | Nausea, vomiting, constipation, confusion, excitement, pulse changes, nasal congestion, flushing, dry mouth. | May cause drowsiness. | Take 30 minutes before meals. | Also used to treat infant colic. |
| **Isopropamide Iodide**<br>*Darbid* tablet (℞) | Nausea, vomiting, constipation, confusion, excitement, pulse changes, nasal congestion, flushing, dry mouth. | May cause drowsiness. | Take 30 minutes before meals. | Used only for the treatment of peptic ulcer. |
| **Metoclopramide**<br>*Reglan* tablet, syrup (℞) | Nausea, diarrhea, restlessness, fatigue, weakness, depression, increased blood pressure, impaired vision. | May cause drowsiness. Consult a physician if involuntary movement of eyes, face, or limbs occurs. | Take 30 minutes before meals. | Used to treat nausea and vomiting from chemotherapy, gastroesophageal reflux, anorexia nervosa, and esophageal bleeding. |
| **Oxyphencyclimine HCl**<br>*Daricon* tablet (℞) | Nausea, vomiting, constipation, confusion, excitement, pulse changes, nasal congestion, flushing, dry mouth. | May cause drowsiness. | Take 30 minutes before meals. | |

**ACTION** These drugs typically slow the activity of the stomach and intestine, reduce cramping, reduce secretions, and relax the urinary bladder. They also may slow or increase the heart rate, block sweating, which may increase body temperature, and dilate the pupils of the eyes.

**INDICATION** As a group these medications may be used for peptic ulcers, diarrhea, colic, urinary problems, and motion sickness, as well as other disorders.

| Generic Name<br>*Brand Name* | Side Effects | Warnings | Dosing | Notes |
|---|---|---|---|---|
| **Propantheline Bromide**<br>*Pro-Banthine*<br>tablet (℞) | Nausea, vomiting, constipation, confusion, excitement, pulse changes, nasal congestion, flushing, dry mouth. | May cause drowsiness. | Take 30 minutes before meals. | |

Gastrointestinal & Urinary

## Antidiarrheals

**ACTION** Antidiarrheals work by several different methods. Some decrease or reduce intestinal movement, while others cause fluid absorption, modify intestinal bacteria, or reduce inflammation.

**INDICATION** Treatment of diarrhea.

| Generic Name<br>*Brand Name* | Side Effects | Warnings | Dosing | Notes |
|---|---|---|---|---|
| **Activated Attapulgite**<br>*Diasorb* tablet, liquid (OTC) | Constipation, nausea, vomiting. | | | Works as an adsorbent. |
| **Attapulgite**<br>*Kaopectate Advanced Formula, Donnagel*<br>suspension (OTC) | Constipation, nausea, vomiting. | | | Works as an adsorbent. |
| **Bismuth Subsalicylate**<br>*Pepto-Bismol*<br>tablet, suspension (OTC) | Constipation, darkening of the tongue and stools. | May cause stool to turn gray-black. Do not swallow tablets whole. | Shake liquid well. | Also used to treat nausea, stomach cramps, and to prevent "traveler's diarrhea." |

**ACTION** Antidiarrheals work by several different methods. Some decrease or reduce intestinal movement, while others cause fluid absorption, modify intestinal bacteria, or reduce inflammation.

**INDICATION** Treatment of diarrhea.

| Generic Name<br>*Brand Name* | Side Effects | Warnings | Dosing | Notes |
|---|---|---|---|---|
| **Difenoxin HCl,**<br>**Atropine Sulfate**<br>*Motofen* tablet<br>(℞, C-IV) | Nausea, vomiting, dry mouth, flushing, blurred vision, constipation. | Avoid alcohol and other sedatives that can cause drowsiness. | | |
| **Diphenoxylate**<br>**with Atropine**<br>**Sulfate**<br>*Lomotil, Lonox*<br>tablet, liquid<br>(℞, C-V) | Nausea, vomiting, dry mouth, flushing, blurred vision, constipation. | Avoid alcohol and other sedatives that can cause drowsiness. | | |
| **Lactobacillus**<br>*Bacid, Lactinex*<br>tablet, capsule,<br>granules (OTC) | | | May need to be refrigerated. | Used to create a more normal bacterial state in the digestive tract, including diarrhea resulting from antibiotic use. |
| **Loperamide HCl**<br>*Imodium A-D*<br>tablet, liquid (OTC)<br>*Imodium* capsule<br>(℞) | Constipation, nausea, dry mouth, fever. | May cause drowsiness or dizziness. Use caution when alertness required. | | |

## Antiflatulents

**ACTION** Relieves flatulence by either dispersing and preventing formation of gas pockets or by reducing the volume of gas within the GI tract.

**INDICATION** Relief of abdominal discomfort, gas pain, and flatulence due to air or gases in the stomach or intestines.

| Generic Name<br>*Brand Name* | Side Effects | Warnings | Dosing | Notes |
|---|---|---|---|---|
| **Charcoal**<br>*Charcocaps*<br>capsule (OTC) | Diarrhea | Consult a physician if diarrhea continues for more than 2 days. | Take 2 hours before or 1 hour after other medications. | |
| **Charcoal,**<br>**Simetecone**<br>*Flatulex* tablet<br>(OTC) | Diarrhea | Consult a physician if diarrhea continues for more than 2 days. | Take 2 hours before or 1 hour after other medications. | |
| **Simethicone**<br>*Mylicon,*<br>*Phazyme, Gas-X*<br>tablet, liquid<br>(OTC) | | | Take after meals and at bedtime. | |

## Antiulcer Agents

**ACTION** Antiulcer agents work by blocking or reducing the amount of acid secreted by the stomach.

**INDICATION** Used for heartburn, acid indigestion, sour stomach, stomach ulcers, and duodenal ulcers. Some are used to treat gastroesophageal reflux.

| Generic Name<br>*Brand Name* | Side Effects | Warnings | Dosing | Notes |
|---|---|---|---|---|
| **Cisapride**<br>*Propulsid* tablet,<br>suspension (℞) | Stomach pain, constipation, nausea, gas, headache, runny nose, body pain, fever, abnormal vision. | Use with alcohol or other depressants will intensify drowsiness. | Take before meals. | Used to treat nighttime heartburn. |

Gastrointestinal & Urinary

**ACTION** Antiulcer agents work by blocking or reducing the amount of acid secreted by the stomach.

**INDICATION** Used for heartburn, acid indigestion, sour stomach, stomach ulcers, and duodenal ulcers. Some are used to treat gastroesophageal reflux.

| Generic Name<br>*Brand Name* | Side Effects | Warnings | Dosing | Notes |
|---|---|---|---|---|
| **Lansoprazole**<br>*Prevacid*<br>capsule (℞) | Diarrhea, nausea, stomach pain, headache, dizziness, difficult breathing. | | Take at least 1 hour before eating. | Antacids can be used while on this medication. |
| **Misoprostol**<br>*Cytotec* tablet (℞) | Nausea, vomiting, diarrhea, constipation, gas, vaginal bleeding, painful menstruation. | Avoid magnesium-containing antacids. Do not take for longer than 2 weeks except under the advice of a doctor. | May take after a meal to reduce diarrhea. | To prevent formation of ulcers when taking an NSAID or aspirin. |
| **Omeprazole**<br>*Prilosec* capsule<br>(℞) | Nausea, vomiting, diarrhea, stomach pain, dizziness, weakness, headache, back pain. | | Take at least 1 hour before a meal. | Short-term treatment of duodenal ulcers. Antacids can be used with this medication. |
| **Sucralfate**<br>*Carafate* tablet,<br>suspension (℞) | Diarrhea, constipation, nausea, dry mouth, dizziness. | Avoid antacids within 30 minutes before or after Sucralfate. | Take on an empty stomach 1 hour before meal. | Forms a protective layer on the ulcer to serve as a barrier to the acid. May be used for oral and esophageal ulcers. |

# H$_2$-Antagonists

**ACTION** Inhibit gastric acid secretion in the stomach. Treatment failure with one H$_2$-antagonist probably indicates that none of the H$_2$-antagonists will work.

**INDICATION** Used for heartburn, acid indigestion, sour stomach, stomach ulcers, and duodenal ulcers. Some are used to treat gastroesophageal reflux.

| Generic Name<br>Brand Name | Side Effects | Warnings | Dosing | Notes |
|---|---|---|---|---|
| **Cimetidine**<br>*Tagamet HB*<br>  tablet (OTC)<br>*Tagamet* tablet,<br>  liquid (℞) | Nausea, vomiting, diarrhea, constipation, confusion, depression, fatigue, dizziness. | Avoid alcohol while taking this medication. | May take without regard to meals. | May be used to treat certain viral infections. OTC dose—Do not take for longer than 2 weeks except under the advice of a doctor. |
| **Famotidine**<br>*Pepcid AC* tablet<br>  (OTC)<br>*Pepcid* tablet,<br>  suspension (℞) | Nausea, vomiting, diarrhea, constipation, confusion, depression, fatigue, dizziness. | Avoid alcohol while taking this medication. | May take without regard to meals. | OTC dose—Do not take for longer than 2 weeks except under the advice of a doctor. |
| **Nizatidine**<br>*Axid AR* tablet<br>  (OTC)<br>*Axid* capsule (℞) | Nausea, vomiting, diarrhea, constipation, confusion, depression, fatigue, dizziness. | Avoid alcohol while taking this medication. | May take without regard to meals. | May be used to treat certain viral infections. OTC dose—Do not take for longer than 2 weeks except under the advice of a doctor. |
| **Ranitidine**<br>*Zantac 75* tablet<br>  (OTC)<br>*Zantac* tablet,<br>  capsule, syrup (℞) | Nausea, vomiting, diarrhea, constipation, confusion, depression, fatigue, dizziness. | Avoid alcohol while taking this medication. | May take without regard to meals. | OTC dose—Do not take for longer than 2 weeks except under the advice of a doctor. |

Gastrointestinal & Urinary

## Laxatives—Stimulants

**ACTION** Stimulant laxatives promote bowel emptying by direct action on intestinal mucosa, by stimulating the myenteric plexus, and by altering water and electrolyte secretion.

**INDICATION** Short-term treatment of constipation. Before using laxatives, consider other factors affecting bowel function such as diet, medication use, sufficient fluid intake, roughage, and daily exercise, which can affect or prevent constipation. Chronic use of laxatives can result in physical dependence.

| Generic Name<br>*Brand Name* | Side Effects | Warnings | Dosing | Notes |
|---|---|---|---|---|
| **Bisacodyl**<br>*Dulcolax* tablet,<br>suppository (OTC) | Nausea, vomiting, stomachache, bowel cramping, dizziness, sweating. | Do not crush tablets. | Take with a full glass of water or juice. | Effects generally take 6 to 10 hours to occur. |
| **Casanthranol,<br>Docusate**<br>*Peri-Colace,<br>Dialose Plus* capsule, liquid (OTC) | Nausea, vomiting, stomachache, bowel cramping, diarrhea. | | Take with a full glass of water or juice. | Works by softening the feces and irritating intestinal tract. |
| **Castor Oil**<br>*Neoloid* emulsion (OTC) | Nausea, vomiting, stomachache, bowel cramping, dizziness, sweating. | | Take with a full glass of water or juice. | Effects generally take 2 to 6 hours to occur. |
| **Phenolphthalein**<br>*Alophen,<br>Feen-a-Mint,<br>Ex-Lax* tablet (OTC) | Nausea, vomiting, stomachache, bowel cramping, dizziness, sweating, discoloration of the urine | **All products containing this ingredient were removed from the market in 1997.** | Take with a full glass of water or juice. | Effects generally take 6 to 10 hours to occur. |
| **Senna**<br>*Senokot, Black-Draught,<br>Fletcher's Castoria* tablet, liquid (OTC) | Nausea, vomiting, stomachache, bowel cramping, dizziness, sweating. | | Take with a full glass of water or juice. | Effects generally take 6 to 10 hours to occur. |

# Laxatives—Others

**ACTION** Laxatives promote bowel emptying. Some work by holding water and swell in the intestines, which stimulates intestinal activity. Stool softeners work by mixing fat and water into fecal matter, which softens the stool.

**INDICATION** Short-term treatment of constipation. Before using laxatives consider other factors affecting bowel function such as diet, medication use, sufficient fluid intake, roughage, and daily exercise, which can affect or prevent constipation. Chronic use of laxatives can result in physical dependence.

| Generic Name<br>*Brand Name* | Side Effects | Warnings | Dosing | Notes |
|---|---|---|---|---|
| **Docusate**<br>**Calcium**<br>*Surfak* capsule<br>(OTC) | Nausea, vomiting, stomachache, bowel cramping, diarrhea. | | Take with a full glass of water or juice. | Works by softening the feces. Effects generally take 24 to 72 hours to occur. |
| **Docusate**<br>**Potassium**<br>*Dialose* capsule<br>(OTC) | Nausea, vomiting, stomachache, bowel cramping, diarrhea. | | Take with a full glass of water or juice. | Works by softening the feces. Effects generally take 24 to 72 hours to occur. |
| **Docusate**<br>**Sodium**<br>*Colace* capsule,<br>syrup, liquid<br>(OTC) | Nausea, vomiting, stomachache, bowel cramping, diarrhea. | | Take with a full glass of water or juice. | Works by softening the feces. Effects generally take 24 to 72 hours to occur. |
| **Glycerin**<br>*Glycerin*<br>suppository (OTC) | Rectal bleeding, bowel cramping, muscle cramps. | Do not use if experiencing abdominal pain, nausea, or vomiting. | | Glycerin irritates the colon to stimulate bowel movements. Effects usually occur in 30 minutes. |
| **Lactulose**<br>*Cephulac,*<br>*Chronulac* syrup<br>(℞) | Gas, belching, stomach pain, bowel cramping, nausea, vomiting, diarrhea. | Do not take other laxatives while using Lactulose. | May be mixed with juice, water, or milk. | Also used for certain liver diseases. |

Gastrointestinal & Urinary

**ACTION** Laxatives promote bowel emptying. Some work by holding water and swell in the intestines, which stimulates intestinal activity. Stool softeners work by mixing fat and water into fecal matter, which softens the stool.

**INDICATION** Short-term treatment of constipation. Before using laxatives consider other factors affecting bowel function such as diet, medication use, sufficient fluid intake, roughage, and daily exercise, which can affect or prevent constipation. Chronic use of laxatives can result in physical dependence.

| Generic Name<br>*Brand Name* | Side Effects | Warnings | Dosing | Notes |
|---|---|---|---|---|
| **Magnesium Citrate**<br>*Citroma, Citrate of Magnesia* liquid (OTC) | Feeling of fullness, bowel cramping. | Do not use if experiencing nausea, vomiting, or abdominal pain. | Take with a full glass of water or juice. | Causes water to accumulate in the intestines. Used to clean the bowels prior to surgery. Effects generally take 3 to 6 hours to occur. |
| **Methylcellulose**<br>*Citrucel* powder (OTC) | Feeling of fullness, bowel cramping. | Do not use if experiencing nausea, vomiting, or abdominal pain. | Take with a full glass of water or juice. | As a bulk-producing treatment can also be used to treat diarrhea. Effects generally take 12 to 24 hours to occur, but may take up to 72 hours. |
| **Mineral Oil**<br>*Agoral, Kondremul* emulsion (OTC) | Nausea, vomiting, bowel cramping, diarrhea, weakness, rectal bleeding, sweating. | May reduce absorption of fat-soluble vitamins. | Take with a full glass of water or juice on empty stomach. | Lubricates intestines and softens feces. Effects generally take 6 to 8 hours to occur. |

**ACTION** Laxatives promote bowel emptying. Some work by holding water and swell in the intestines, which stimulates intestinal activity. Stool softeners work by mixing fat and water into fecal matter, which softens the stool.

**INDICATION** Short-term treatment of constipation. Before using laxatives consider other factors affecting bowel function such as diet, medication use, sufficient fluid intake, roughage, and daily exercise, which can affect or prevent constipation. Chronic use of laxatives can result in physical dependence.

| Generic Name Brand Name | Side Effects | Warnings | Dosing | Notes |
|---|---|---|---|---|
| **Polycarbophil** FiberCon, Mitrolan tablet (OTC) | Feeling of fullness, bowel cramping. | Do not use if experiencing nausea, vomiting, or abdominal pain. | Take with a full glass of water or juice. | As a bulk-producing treatment can also be used to treat diarrhea. Also used to treat diverticulitis. Effects generally take 12 to 24 hours to occur, but may take up to 72 hours. |
| **Psyllium** Hydrocil, Konsyl, Metamucil, Perdiem powder (OTC) | Feeling of fullness, bowel cramping. | Do not use if experiencing nausea, vomiting, or abdominal pain. | Take with a full glass of water or juice. | As a bulk-producing treatment can also be used to treat diarrhea. Also used to treat irritable bowel syndrome. Effects generally take 12 to 24 hours to occur, but may take up to 72 hours. |

Gastrointestinal & Urinary

# Urinary Acidifiers

**ACTION** To acidify the urine and to lower urinary calcium concentrations.

**INDICATION** To lower the urinary pH, which can increase antibacterial effect of certain urinary tract medications.

| Generic Name<br>*Brand Name* | Side Effects | Warnings | Dosing | Notes |
|---|---|---|---|---|
| **Ammonium Chloride**<br>*Ammonium Chloride* tablet (OTC) | Gastric irritation, nausea, vomiting. | Tablets should be soaked and dissolved in water before taking. | Take with plenty of water. Take with meals and at bedtime. | |
| **Potassium Acid Phosphate**<br>*K-Phos* tablets (℞) | Abdominal discomfort, diarrhea, nausea, vomiting. | | Take with plenty of water. | |

# Urinary Alkalinizers

**ACTION** Increases the excretion of free base in the urine, which increases the urinary pH.

**INDICATION** To correct acidosis in renal disorders and to minimize uric acid crystallization in gout.

| Generic Name<br>*Brand Name* | Side Effects | Warnings | Dosing | Notes |
|---|---|---|---|---|
| **Sodium Citrate**<br>*Bicitra* solution (℞) | Diarrhea, nausea. | Notify physician if stomach pain, vomiting, or convulsions occurs. | Take with water. Take after meals to minimize laxative effect. | |
| **Potassium Citrate**<br>*Urocit-K* tablet (℞) | Nausea, vomiting, diarrhea, edema, high blood pressure, weakness. | | Take after meals. Take with water and follow with more water. | |

# Urinary Analgesics

**ACTION** Excreted in the urine where a topical analgesic effect on the urinary tract mucosa occurs.

**INDICATION** Relief of pain, burning, and urinary urgency.

| Generic Name Brand Name | Side Effects | Warnings | Dosing | Notes |
|---|---|---|---|---|
| **Pentosan Polysulfate Sodium** *Elmiron* capsule (℞) | Headache, depression, alopecia, rash, nausea, vomiting. | May increase bleeding time. | Take with water 1 hour before or 2 hours after meals. | |
| **Phenazopyridine HCl** *Azo-Standard* tablet (OTC) *Pyridium*, *Urogesic* tablet (℞) | Headache, reddish-orange urine, rash, itching. | Take with food to avoid stomach upset. | | Do not use for more than 2 to 3 days for infection. |

Gastrointestinal & Urinary

# Urinary Tract Products

**ACTION** These drugs typically slow the activity of the stomach and intestine, and reduce cramping, reduce secretions, and relax the urinary bladder. They also may slow or increase the heart rate, block sweating, which may increase body temperature, and dilate the pupils of the eyes.

**INDICATION** As a group, these medications may be used for peptic ulcers, diarrhea, colic, urinary problems, motion sickness, and other disorders.

| Generic Name Brand Name | Side Effects | Warnings | Dosing | Notes |
|---|---|---|---|---|
| **Bethanechol Chloride** *Duvoid*, *Urecholine* tablet (℞) | Salivation, sweating, flushing, dizziness. | | Take on an empty stomach. | Used to cause urination by stimulating bladder contraction. |
| **Flavoxate HCl** *Urispas* tablet (℞) | Nausea, vomiting, vertigo, dizziness, dry mouth, increased heart rate. | May cause drowsiness. Use caution when performing tasks that require alertness. | | Used to prevent painful urination, frequency, urgency, and incontinence. |

**ACTION** These drugs typically slow the activity of the stomach and intestine, and reduce cramping, reduce secretions, and relax the urinary bladder. They also may slow or increase the heart rate, block sweating, which may increase body temperature, and dilate the pupils of the eyes.

**INDICATION** As a group, these medications may be used for peptic ulcers, diarrhea, colic, urinary problems, motion sickness, and other disorders.

| Generic Name<br>*Brand Name* | Side Effects | Warnings | Dosing | Notes |
|---|---|---|---|---|
| **Oxybutynin Chloride**<br>*Ditropan* tablet, syrup (℞) | Nausea, vomiting, constipation, weakness, rapid heart rate, vision problems. | May cause drowsiness. Use caution when performing tasks that require alertness. | | Used to prevent frequent or painful urination and incontinence. |

# Anti-Infective Agents

## Anthelmintics

**ACTION** Each medication works by either killing or halting the growth of the parasite.

**INDICATION** Each medication works for specific types of parasitic intestinal and tissue nematodes.

| Generic Name *Brand Name* | Side Effects | Warnings | Dosing | Notes |
|---|---|---|---|---|
| **Mebendazole** *Vermox* chewable tablet (℞) | Stomachache, diarrhea, fever. | To prevent reinfection, disinfect toilet and wash all bed linens, towels, and nightclothes daily. | Chew or crush tablet with food. | Effective against pinworm, roundworm, hookworm, and whipworm infections. |
| **Piperazine** *Vermizine* tablet, syrup (℞) | Nausea, vomiting, headache, vertigo, blurred vision. | To prevent reinfection, disinfect toilet and wash all bed linens, towels, and nightclothes daily. | Take on an empty stomach. | Effective for pinworm and roundworm infections. |
| **Pyrantel** *Antiminth* suspension (℞) *Pin-Rid, Reese's Pinworm* liquid (OTC) | Nausea, vomiting, diarrhea, dizziness, sleeplessness. | To prevent reinfection, disinfect toilet and wash all bed linens, towels, and nightclothes daily. | May be taken regardless of food. | Effective for pinworm and roundworm infections. |
| **Thiabendazole** *Mintezol* chewable tablet, suspension (℞) | Appetite loss, nausea, diarrhea, dizziness, fever. | To prevent reinfection, disinfect toilet and wash all bed linens, towels, and nightclothes daily. | Chew tablet. Take with food. | Effective for pinworm, threadworm, round worm, hookworm, and whipworm infections. |

# Antibiotic—Cephalosporins

**ACTION** Cephalosporin antibiotics kill bacteria by preventing the formation of the normal cell bacterial wall, increasing the likelihood that the cell will rupture. Allergic reactions include mild itching, rash, fever, joint pain, chest tightness, difficult breathing, and chills, and should be reported to a physician. A history of previous allergies to penicillins or other cephalosporins increases the risk of allergic reaction. Cephalosporins may interfere with urine tests for glucose.

**INDICATION** Used to treat infections caused by bacteria. It is important to take the full course of therapy to prevent a recurrence of the infection.

| Generic Name<br>Brand Name | Side Effects | Warnings | Dosing | Notes |
|---|---|---|---|---|
| **Cefaclor**<br>*Ceclor* capsule,<br>suspension (℞) | Nausea, vomiting, diarrhea, indigestion, gas, headache, confusion, flushing, sweating, low blood pressure, edema. | | May be taken with food or milk to prevent stomach upset. | Store suspension in the refrigerator. |
| **Cefadroxil**<br>*Duricef* tablet,<br>capsule, suspension (℞) | Nausea, vomiting, diarrhea, indigestion, gas, headache, confusion, flushing, sweating, low blood pressure, edema. | | May be taken with food or milk to prevent stomach upset. | Store suspension in the refrigerator. |
| **Ceftibuten**<br>*Cedax* capsule,<br>suspension (℞) | Nausea, vomiting, diarrhea, indigestion, gas, headache, confusion, flushing, sweating, low blood pressure, edema. | | May be taken with food or milk to prevent stomach upset. | Store suspension in the refrigerator. |
| **Cefixime**<br>*Suprax* tablet,<br>suspension (℞) | Nausea, vomiting, diarrhea, indigestion, gas, headache, confusion, flushing, sweating, low blood pressure, edema. | | May be taken with food or milk to prevent stomach upset. | Store suspension at room temperature. |

**ACTION** Cephalosporin antibiotics kill bacteria by preventing the formation of the normal cell bacterial wall, increasing the likelihood that the cell will rupture. Allergic reactions include mild itching, rash, fever, joint pain, chest tightness, difficult breathing, and chills, and should be reported to a physician. A history of previous allergies to penicillins or other cephalosporins increases the risk of allergic reaction. Cephalosporins may interfere with urine tests for glucose.

**INDICATION** Used to treat infections caused by bacteria. It is important to take the full course of therapy to prevent a recurrence of the infection.

| Generic Name Brand Name | Side Effects | Warnings | Dosing | Notes |
|---|---|---|---|---|
| **Cefpodoxime Proxetil** Vantin tablet, suspension (℞) | Nausea, vomiting, diarrhea, indigestion, gas, headache, confusion, flushing, sweating, low blood pressure, edema. | | Take with food to increase absorption. | Store suspension in the refrigerator. |
| **Cefprozil** Cefzil tablet, suspension (℞) | Nausea, vomiting, diarrhea, indigestion, gas, headache, confusion, flushing, sweating, low blood pressure, edema. | | May be taken with food or milk to prevent stomach upset. | Store suspension in the refrigerator. |
| **Cefuroxime** Ceftin tablet, suspension (℞) | Nausea, vomiting, diarrhea, indigestion, gas, headache, confusion, flushing, sweating, low blood pressure, edema. | | Take with food to increase absorption. | Store suspension in the refrigerator or at room temperature. |
| **Cephalexin** Keflex capsule, suspension (℞) Keftab tablet (℞) | Nausea, vomiting, diarrhea, indigestion, gas, headache, confusion, flushing, sweating, low blood pressure, edema. | | May be taken with food or milk to prevent stomach upset. | Store suspension in the refrigerator. |

Anti-Infectives

**ACTION** Cephalosporin antibiotics kill bacteria by preventing the formation of the normal cell bacterial wall, increasing the likelihood that the cell will rupture. Allergic reactions include mild itching, rash, fever, joint pain, chest tightness, difficult breathing, and chills, and should be reported to a physician. A history of previous allergies to penicillins or other cephalosporins increases the risk of allergic reaction. Cephalosporins may interfere with urine tests for glucose.

**INDICATION** Used to treat infections caused by bacteria. It is important to take the full course of therapy to prevent a recurrence of the infection.

| Generic Name<br>*Brand Name* | Side Effects | Warnings | Dosing | Notes |
|---|---|---|---|---|
| **Cephradine**<br>*Velosef* capsule,<br>suspension (℞) | Nausea, vomiting, diarrhea, indigestion, gas, headache, confusion, flushing, sweating, low blood pressure, edema. | | May be taken with food or milk to prevent stomach upset. | Store suspension in the refrigerator. |
| **Loracarbef**<br>*Lorabid* capsule,<br>suspension (℞) | Nausea, vomiting, diarrhea, indigestion, gas, headache, confusion, flushing, sweating, low blood pressure, edema. | | Take at least 1 hour before or 2 hours after eating a meal. | Store suspension at room temperature. |

# Antibiotic—Fluoroquinolones

**ACTION** Fluoroquinolones inhibit DNA production of certain bacteria resulting in cell death. Allergic reactions include rash, facial swelling, and difficult breathing. Patients with a history of seizures or other nervous system disorders may experience tremors, confusion, light-headedness, or restlessness.

**INDICATION** Used to treat infections ranging from lower respiratory disorders, sexually transmitted diseases, skin infections, and urinary tract infections caused by bacteria. It is important to take the full course of therapy to prevent a recurrence of the infection.

| Generic Name<br>*Brand Name* | Side Effects | Warnings | Dosing | Notes |
|---|---|---|---|---|
| **Ciprofloxacin**<br>*Cipro* tablet (℞) | Nausea, vomiting, diarrhea, stomachache, dizziness, headache, restlessness. | Drug may make user sensitive to the sun. | May be taken with or without meals. Do not take with dairy products. Drink plenty of fluids. | Also used for infectious diarrhea and typhoid fever. |
| **Enoxacin**<br>*Penetrex* tablet (℞) | Nausea, vomiting, diarrhea, stomachache, dizziness, headache, indigestion, vertigo, sleeplessness, unusual taste. | Drug may make user sensitive to the sun. Drink plenty of fluids. | Take at least 1 hour before or 2 hours after a meal. Avoid antacids, iron, or zinc products 8 hours before and 2 hours after taking this drug. | Avoid consumption of caffeine. |
| **Levofloxacin**<br>*Levaquin* tablet (℞) | Diarrhea, nausea, flatulence, rash, headache, constipation, insomnia. | Phototoxicity may occur with this drug. Avoid excessive sunlight or UV light. Drink plenty of fluids. | May be taken without regard to meals. Avoid antacids, iron, or zinc products 2 hours before and 2 hours after taking this drug. | |
| **Lomefloxacin HCl**<br>*Maxaquin* tablet (℞) | Nausea, vomiting, diarrhea, stomachache, dizziness, headache. | Drug may make user sensitive to the sun. Drink plenty of fluids. | May be taken with or without meals. | |

Anti-Infectives

**ACTION** Fluoroquinolones inhibit DNA production of certain bacteria resulting in cell death. Allergic reactions include rash, facial swelling, and difficult breathing. Patients with a history of seizures or other nervous system disorders may experience tremors, confusion, light-headedness, or restlessness.

**INDICATION** Used to treat infections ranging from lower respiratory disorders, sexually transmitted diseases, skin infections, and urinary tract infections caused by bacteria. It is important to take the full course of therapy to prevent a recurrence of the infection.

| Generic Name<br>Brand Name | Side Effects | Warnings | Dosing | Notes |
|---|---|---|---|---|
| **Norfloxacin**<br>*Noroxin* tablet (℞) | Nausea, vomiting, diarrhea, stomachache, dizziness, headache, weakness, constipation, gas, drowsiness, dry mouth. | Drug may make user sensitive to the sun. Drink plenty of fluids. | Take on an empty stomach at least 1 hour before or 2 hours after a meal. | |
| **Ofloxacin**<br>*Floxin* tablet (℞) | Nausea, vomiting, diarrhea, stomachache, dizziness, headache, gas, nervousness, lack of energy, dry mouth, chest pain, vaginal irritation. | Drug may make user sensitive to the sun. | Take on an empty stomach. Avoid calcium-containing products within 2 hours of taking this drug. | Also used to treat inflammation of the prostrate. |
| **Sparfloxacin**<br>*Zagam* tablet (℞) | Diarrhea, nausea, headache, dyspepsia, dizziness, insomnia, vomiting, flatulence. | Severe phototoxicity may occur with this drug. Avoid direct or indirect sunlight or UV light during therapy and for 5 days after. Drink plenty of fluids. | May be taken without regard to meals. Avoid antacids, iron, or zinc products for 4 hours after taking this drug. | |

## Antibiotic—Macrolides

**ACTION** Macrolide antibiotics suppress the formation of protein by bacteria, thereby slowing bacterial growth or causing bacteria cell death.

**INDICATION** Used to treat infections caused by bacteria. It is important to take the full course of therapy to prevent a reoccurrence of the infection.

| Generic Name<br>*Brand Name* | Side Effects | Warnings | Dosing | Notes |
|---|---|---|---|---|
| **Azithromycin**<br>*Zithromax* tablet, suspension (℞) | Nausea, stomach pain, vomiting, indigestion, vaginal infections, headache, difficult breathing. | Do not take with food. If diarrhea occurs contact a doctor. May make user sensitive to the sun. | Take suspension 1 hour before or 2 hours after a meal or antacids. | Store suspension in the refrigerator or room temperature. |
| **Clarithromycin**<br>*Biaxin* tablet, suspension (℞) | Nausea, stomach pain, diarrhea, vomiting, indigestion, headache, sleeplessness, dizziness, dark urine. | Contact a physician if hives, itching, or difficult breathing develops. | May be taken with or without food or milk. | Store suspension at room temperature. Do not refrigerate. |
| **Dirithromycin**<br>*Dynabac* tablet (℞) | Nausea, stomach pain, vomiting, indigestion, headache, weakness, difficult breathing. | If diarrhea occurs, contact a doctor. | Take with food or within 1 hour of eating. | |
| **Erythromycin Base**<br>*E-Mycin, Ery-Tab* tablet (℞)<br>*ERYC* capsule (℞) | Nausea, vomiting, appetite loss, diarrhea, jaundice, fever, lack of energy, difficult breathing. | | Take on an empty stomach unless stomach upset occurs; then take with food. | |
| **Erythromycin Estolate**<br>*Ilosone* tablet, capsule, suspension (℞) | Nausea, vomiting, appetite loss, diarrhea, jaundice, fever, lack of energy, difficult breathing. | | Take on an empty stomach unless stomach upset occurs; then take with food. | Store suspension in the refrigerator to maintain taste. |

Anti-Infectives

**ACTION** Macrolide antibiotics suppress the formation of protein by bacteria, thereby slowing bacterial growth or causing bacteria cell death.

**INDICATION** Used to treat infections caused by bacteria. It is important to take the full course of therapy to prevent a reoccurrence of the infection.

| Generic Name<br>*Brand Name* | Side Effects | Warnings | Dosing | Notes |
|---|---|---|---|---|
| **Erythromycin Ethylsuccinate**<br>*E.E.S.* tablet (℞)<br>*E.E.S., Pediamycin, EryPed* suspension (℞) | Nausea, vomiting, appetite loss, diarrhea, jaundice, fever, lack of energy, difficult breathing. | | Take on an empty stomach unless stomach upset occurs; then take with food. | Store suspension in the refrigerator to maintain taste. |
| **Erythromycin Stearate**<br>*Erythrocin* tablet (℞) | Nausea, vomiting, appetite loss, diarrhea, jaundice, fever, lack of energy, difficult breathing. | | Take on an empty stomach unless stomach upset occurs; then take with food. | |
| **Troleandomycin**<br>*Tao* capsule (℞) | Abdominal cramps, nausea, vomiting, diarrhea. | | Take on an empty stomach unless stomach upset occurs; then take with food. | |

# Antibiotic—Penicillins

**ACTION** Penicillins prevent the production of bacteria cell walls and will kill bacteria when a proper concentration of the drug is in the blood, tissue, or other body fluid where the bacteria are located. Allergic reactions to penicillins include wheezing, hives, itching, swelling, difficulty breathing, and joint and muscle pain.

**INDICATION** Used to treat mild to moderate infections for penicillin-sensitive bacteria. It is important to take the full course of therapy to prevent a recurrence of the infection. If an allergic reaction has occurred to one of the penicillin products, then patient is likely to be allergic to all the penicillin products.

| Generic Name<br>*Brand Name* | Side Effects | Warnings | Dosing | Notes |
|---|---|---|---|---|
| **Amoxicillin**<br>*Amoxil, Polymox, Trimox, Wymox*<br>capsules, suspension (℞)<br>*Amoxil* chewable tablet (℞) | Nausea, vomiting, diarrhea, gas, secondary fungal infections, dizziness, low blood pressure. | | May be taken regardless of food. | Store suspension in refrigerator. |
| **Amoxicillin, Clavulanate Potassium**<br>*Augmentin* tablet, chewable tablet, suspension (℞) | Nausea, vomiting, diarrhea, gas, secondary fungal infections, dizziness, low blood pressure. | | May be taken regardless of food. | Store suspension in refrigerator. |
| **Ampicillin**<br>*Amcill, Omnipen, Polycillin, Principen*<br>capsules, suspension (℞) | Nausea, vomiting, diarrhea, gas, secondary fungal infections, dizziness, low blood pressure. | | Take 1 hour before or 2 hours after meals. | Store suspension in refrigerator. |
| **Bacampicillin**<br>*Spectrobid* tablets, suspension (℞) | Nausea, vomiting, diarrhea, gas, secondary fungal infections, dizziness, low blood pressure. | | Take 1 hour before or 2 hours after meals. | Store suspension in refrigerator. |
| **Carbenicillin Indanyl Sodium**<br>*Geocillin* tablet (℞) | Nausea, vomiting, diarrhea, gas, secondary fungal infections, dizziness, low blood pressure. | | Take 1 hour before or 2 hours after meals. | |

Anti-Infectives

**ACTION** Penicillins prevent the production of bacteria cell walls and will kill bacteria when a proper concentration of the drug is in the blood, tissue, or other body fluid where the bacteria are located. Allergic reactions to penicillins include wheezing, hives, itching, swelling, difficulty breathing, and joint and muscle pain.

**INDICATION** Used to treat mild to moderate infections for penicillin-sensitive bacteria. It is important to take the full course of therapy to prevent a recurrence of the infection. If an allergic reaction has occurred to one of the penicillin products, then patient is likely to be allergic to all the penicillin products.

| Generic Name<br>*Brand Name* | Side Effects | Warnings | Dosing | Notes |
|---|---|---|---|---|
| **Cloxacillin Sodium**<br>*Cloxapen, Tegopen*<br>capsule, suspension (℞) | Nausea, vomiting, diarrhea, gas, secondary fungal infections, dizziness, low blood pressure. | | Take 1 hour before or 2 hours after meals. | Store suspension in refrigerator. |
| **Dicloxacillin Sodium**<br>*Dynapen, Pathocil*<br>capsule, suspension (℞) | Nausea, vomiting, diarrhea, gas, secondary fungal infections, dizziness, low blood pressure. | | Take 1 hour before or 2 hours after meals. | Store suspension in refrigerator. |
| **Nafcillin Sodium**<br>*Unipen* capsule, tablet (℞) | Nausea, vomiting, diarrhea, gas, secondary fungal infections, dizziness, low blood pressure. | | Take 1 hour before or 2 hours after meals. | Store solution in refrigerator. |
| **Oxacillin Sodium**<br>*Prostaphlin, Bactocill* capsule, solution (℞) | Nausea, vomiting, diarrhea, gas, secondary fungal infections, dizziness, low blood pressure. | | Take 1 hour before or 2 hours after meals. | Store solution in refrigerator. |
| **Penicillin G Potassium**<br>*Pentids* tablet, solution (℞) | Nausea, vomiting, diarrhea, gas, secondary fungal infections, dizziness, low blood pressure. | | May take with or without food. | Store solution in refrigerator. |

**ACTION** Penicillins prevent the production of bacteria cell walls and will kill bacteria when a proper concentration of the drug is in the blood, tissue, or other body fluid where the bacteria are located. Allergic reactions to penicillins include wheezing, hives, itching, swelling, difficulty breathing, and joint and muscle pain.

**INDICATION** Used to treat mild to moderate infections for penicillin-sensitive bacteria. It is important to take the full course of therapy to prevent a recurrence of the infection. If an allergic reaction has occurred to one of the penicillin products, then patient is likely to be allergic to all the penicillin products.

| Generic Name<br>Brand Name | Side Effects | Warnings | Dosing | Notes |
|---|---|---|---|---|
| **Penicillin V Potassium**<br>Beepen-VK, Pen-Vee K, Veetids, V-Cillin-K, Ledercill VK tablet, solution (℞) | Nausea, vomiting, diarrhea, gas, secondary fungal infections, dizziness, low blood pressure. | | Take 1 hour before or 2 hours after meals. | Store solution in refrigerator. |

## Antibiotic—Sulfonamides

Anti-Infectives

**ACTION** Sulfonamides inhibit use of para-aminobenzoic acid (PABA) by the bacteria, which is an essential component in folic acid production and bacteria function. Avoid large doses of drugs that may acidify the urine (e.g., Vitamin C).

**INDICATION** Used to treat infections caused by bacteria. Sometimes also used for rheumatoid arthritis, colitis, and Crohn's disease. It is important to take the full course of therapy to prevent a recurrence of the infection.

| Generic Name<br>Brand Name | Side Effects | Warnings | Dosing | Notes |
|---|---|---|---|---|
| **Sulfacytine**<br>Renoquid tablet (℞) | Nausea, vomiting, diarrhea, headache, vertigo, depression, sleeplessness. | Contact a doctor if blood in the urine, easy bruising, ringing in the ears, difficult breathing, fever, or chills develop. Avoid prolonged exposure to the sun as the medication may make user more sensitive to light. | Take on an empty stomach with a full glass of water. | |

**ACTION** Sulfonamides inhibit use of para-aminobenzoic acid (PABA) by the bacteria, which is an essential component in folic acid production and bacteria function. Avoid large doses of drugs that may acidify the urine (e.g., Vitamin C).

**INDICATION** Used to treat infections caused by bacteria. Sometimes also used for rheumatoid arthritis, colitis, and Crohn's disease. It is important to take the full course of therapy to prevent a recurrence of the infection.

| Generic Name<br>*Brand Name* | Side Effects | Warnings | Dosing | Notes |
|---|---|---|---|---|
| **Sulfamethizole**<br>*Thiosulfil Forte*<br>tablet (℞) | Nausea, vomiting, diarrhea, headache, vertigo, depression, sleeplessness. | Contact a doctor if blood in the urine, easy bruising, ringing in the ears, difficult breathing, fever, or chills develop. Avoid prolonged exposure to the sun as the medication may make user more sensitive to light. | Take on an empty stomach with a full glass of water. | |
| **Sulfamethizole, Oxytetracycline, Phenazopyridine**<br>*Urobiotic* capsule<br>(℞) | Nausea, vomiting, diarrhea, headache, vertigo, depression, sleeplessness. | Contact a doctor if blood in the urine, easy bruising, ringing in the ears, difficult breathing, fever, or chills develop. Avoid prolonged exposure to the sun as the medication may make user more sensitive to light. | Take on an empty stomach with a full glass of water. | Commonly used for urinary tract infections. |

**ACTION** Sulfonamides inhibit use of para-aminobenzoic acid (PABA) by the bacteria, which is an essential component in folic acid production and bacteria function. Avoid large doses of drugs that may acidify the urine (e.g., Vitamin C).

**INDICATION** Used to treat infections caused by bacteria. Sometimes also used for rheumatoid arthritis, colitis, and Crohn's disease. It is important to take the full course of therapy to prevent a recurrence of the infection.

| Generic Name<br>*Brand Name* | Side Effects | Warnings | Dosing | Notes |
|---|---|---|---|---|
| **Sulfamethoxa-<br>zole**<br>*Gantanol* tablet,<br>suspension (℞) | Nausea, vomit-<br>ing, diarrhea,<br>headache, ver-<br>tigo, depression,<br>sleeplessness. | Contact a doctor<br>if blood in the<br>urine, easy<br>bruising, ringing<br>in the ears, dif-<br>ficult breathing,<br>fever, or chills<br>develop. Avoid<br>prolonged expo-<br>sure to the sun<br>as the medica-<br>tion may make<br>user more sensi-<br>tive to light. | Take on an<br>empty stomach<br>with a full glass<br>of water. Shake<br>suspension well<br>before using. | |
| **Sulfamethoxa-<br>zole,<br>Trimethoprim**<br>*TMP-SMZ, Bactrim,<br>Septra, Cotrim*<br>tablet, suspen-<br>sion (℞) | Nausea, vomit-<br>ing, diarrhea,<br>headache, ver-<br>tigo, depression,<br>sleeplessness. | Contact a doctor<br>if blood in the<br>urine, easy<br>bruising, ringing<br>in the ears, dif-<br>ficult breathing,<br>fever, or chills<br>develop. Avoid<br>prolonged expo-<br>sure to the sun<br>as the medica-<br>tion may make<br>user more sensi-<br>tive to light. | Take on an<br>empty stomach<br>with a full glass<br>of water. If<br>stomach upset<br>occurs, take<br>with food. | |

Anti-Infectives

**ACTION** Sulfonamides inhibit use of para-aminobenzoic acid (PABA) by the bacteria, which is an essential component in folic acid production and bacteria function. Avoid large doses of drugs that may acidify the urine (e.g., Vitamin C).

**INDICATION** Used to treat infections caused by bacteria. Sometimes also used for rheumatoid arthritis, colitis, and Crohn's disease. It is important to take the full course of therapy to prevent a recurrence of the infection.

| Generic Name<br>*Brand Name* | Side Effects | Warnings | Dosing | Notes |
|---|---|---|---|---|
| **Sulfasalazine**<br>*Azulfidine,*<br>*Azulfidine EN-tabs*<br>tablet, suspension (℞) | Nausea, vomiting, diarrhea, headache, vertigo, depression, sleeplessness, orange-yellow discoloration of urine. | Contact a doctor if blood in the urine, easy bruising, ringing in the ears, difficult breathing, fever, or chills develop. Avoid prolonged exposure to the sun as the medication may make user more sensitive to light. | Take on an empty stomach with a full glass of water. If stomach upset occurs, take with food. Shake suspension well before using. | |
| **Sulfisoxazole**<br>*Gantrisin* tablet,<br>syrup, suspension (℞) | Nausea, vomiting, diarrhea, headache, vertigo, depression, sleeplessness. | Contact a doctor if blood in the urine, easy bruising, ringing in the ears, difficult breathing, fever, or chills develop. Avoid prolonged exposure to the sun as the medication may make user more sensitive to light. | Take on an empty stomach with a full glass of water. Shake suspension well before using. | |

**ACTION** Sulfonamides inhibit use of para-aminobenzoic acid (PABA) by the bacteria, which is an essential component in folic acid production and bacteria function. Avoid large doses of drugs that may acidify the urine (e.g., Vitamin C).

**INDICATION** Used to treat infections caused by bacteria. Sometimes also used for rheumatoid arthritis, colitis, and Crohn's disease. It is important to take the full course of therapy to prevent a recurrence of the infection.

| Generic Name<br>*Brand Name* | Side Effects | Warnings | Dosing | Notes |
|---|---|---|---|---|
| **Sulfisoxazole,**<br>**Erythromycin**<br>  **Ethylsuccinate**<br>*Pediazole* suspen-<br>  sion (℞) | Nausea, vomit-<br>ing, diarrhea,<br>headache, ver-<br>tigo, depression,<br>sleeplessness. | Contact a doctor<br>if blood in the<br>urine, easy<br>bruising, ringing<br>in the ears, dif-<br>ficult breathing,<br>fever, or chills<br>develop. Avoid<br>prolonged expo-<br>sure to the sun<br>as the medica-<br>tion may make<br>user more sensi-<br>tive to light. | Take with meals<br>or on an empty<br>stomach with a<br>full glass of<br>water. | Commonly used<br>to treat otitis<br>media in<br>children.<br>Refrigerate<br>suspension. |

Anti-Infectives

## Antibiotic—Tetracyclines

**ACTION** Tetracyclines inhibit bacteria's production of protein, which slows and prevents growth and reproduction. Tetracyclines can cause permanent discoloration and inadequate hardening of teeth during tooth development and should not be used during pregnancy or in children under 8. Do not use if medication is outdated as tetracyclines can be toxic to kidneys.

**INDICATION** Used to treat a wide variety of infections susceptible to tetracyclines. Used to treat acne. Tetracyclines can increase sensitivity to the sun. Exposure to the sun should be reduced and sun screens should be used to avoid reaction to the sun.

| Generic Name<br>Brand Name | Side Effects | Warnings | Dosing | Notes |
|---|---|---|---|---|
| **Demeclocycline**<br>*Declomycin*<br>capsule, tablet<br>(Ŗ) | Weakness, excessive thirst, nausea, vomiting, diarrhea, joint pain, anemia, headache, mouth sores. | May cause sensitivity to light. | Take on an empty stomach 1 hour before or 2 hours after a meal and with a full glass of water or other fluid. | Avoid use within 2 to 3 hours of antacids, laxatives, dairy products, and iron-containing products |
| **Doxycycline**<br>*Vibramycin,*<br>*Doryx* capsule (Ŗ)<br>*Vibra-tabs* tablets<br>(Ŗ)<br>*Vibramycin* syrup,<br>suspension (Ŗ) | Nausea, vomiting, diarrhea, joint pain, anemia, headache, mouth sores. | May cause sensitivity to light. | May take with or without food. | Used to prevent "traveler's diarrhea" and for treatment of early Lyme disease. |
| **Methacycline**<br>*Rondomycin*<br>capsule (Ŗ) | Nausea, vomiting, diarrhea, joint pain, anemia, headache, mouth sores. | May cause sensitivity to light. | Take on an empty stomach 1 hour before or 2 hours after a meal and with a full glass of water or other fluid. | Avoid use within 2 to 3 hours of antacids, laxatives, dairy products, and iron-containing products. Recommended for early Lyme disease. |
| **Minocycline**<br>*Minocin* capsule,<br>tablet, suspension<br>(Ŗ) | Nausea, vomiting, diarrhea, joint pain, anemia, headache, mouth sores. | May cause sensitivity to light. | May take with or without food. | Store suspension in the refrigerator. |

**ACTION** Tetracyclines inhibit bacteria's production of protein, which slows and prevents growth and reproduction. Tetracyclines can cause permanent discoloration and inadequate hardening of teeth during tooth development and should not be used during pregnancy or in children under 8. Do not use if medication is outdated as tetracyclines can be toxic to kidneys.

**INDICATION** Used to treat a wide variety of infections susceptible to tetracyclines. Used to treat acne. Tetracyclines can increase sensitivity to the sun. Exposure to the sun should be reduced and sun screens should be used to avoid reaction to the sun.

| Generic Name Brand Name | Side Effects | Warnings | Dosing | Notes |
|---|---|---|---|---|
| **Oxytetracycline** *Terramycin* capsule (R) | Nausea, vomiting, diarrhea, joint pain, anemia, headache, mouth sores. | May cause sensitivity to light. | Take on an empty stomach 1 hour before or 2 hours after a meal and with a full glass of water or other fluid. | Avoid use within 2 to 3 hours of antacids, laxatives, dairy products, and iron-containing products. |
| **Tetracycline** *Achromycin V, Panmycin, Sumycin* capsule, suspension (R) | Nausea, vomiting, diarrhea, joint pain, anemia, headache, mouth sores. | May cause sensitivity to light. | Take on an empty stomach 1 hour before or 2 hours after a meal and with a full glass of water or other fluid. | Avoid use within 2 to 3 hours of antacids, laxatives, dairy products, and iron-containing products. Recommended for early Lyme disease. |

Anti-Infectives

## Antibiotics—Miscellaneous

**ACTION** Antibiotics kill bacteria by preventing the formation of the normal cell bacterial wall increasing the likelihood that the cell will rupture. Allergic reactions include mild itching, rash, fever, joint pain, chest tightness, difficult breathing, and chills, and should be reported to your physician.

**INDICATION** Used to treat infections caused by bacteria. It is important to take the full course of therapy to prevent a reoccurrence of the infection.

| Generic Name Brand Name | Side Effects | Warnings | Dosing | Notes |
|---|---|---|---|---|
| **Atovaquone** *Mepron* suspension (℞) | Nausea, diarrhea, stomach pain, constipation, low blood sugar, low blood pressure. | | Take with meals. | Used to treat *Pneumonitis carinii* pneumonia. |
| **Chloramphenicol** *Chloromycetin* capsule (℞) | Nausea, vomiting, diarrhea, blood disorders, fever, depression. | Contact a doctor if fever, sore throat, unusual bleeding or bruising, diarrhea, or visual disturbances develop. | Take on an empty stomach; however, may be taken with food if stomach upset occurs. | Used to treat acute typhoid fever infection and in cystic fibrosis patients. |
| **Clindamycin** *Cleocin* capsule (℞) | Nausea, vomiting, diarrhea, bloody stools, flaking skin, vaginal infection, sore throat, unpleasant taste. | Notify a doctor if severe diarrhea, bloody stools, or unusual bleeding occurs. | May take without regard to food. | |
| **Fosfomycin Tromethamine** *Monurol* powder (℞) | Diarrhea, vaginitis, nausea, headache, dizziness, dyspepsia, rhinitis, back pain. | If symptoms do not improve within 2 to 3 days, contact a physician. | Can take without regard to meals. Mix medication with 4 ounces of water, stir, and take immediately. | |
| **Kanamycin Sulfate** *Kantrex* capsule (℞) | Nausea, vomiting, diarrhea, dizziness. | Notify a doctor if ringing in the ears or problems urinating develop. | Drink plenty of fluids. | Used to treat hepatic coma. |

**ACTION** Antibiotics kill bacteria by preventing the formation of the normal cell bacterial wall increasing the likelihood that the cell will rupture. Allergic reactions include mild itching, rash, fever, joint pain, chest tightness, difficult breathing, and chills, and should be reported to your physician.

**INDICATION** Used to treat infections caused by bacteria. It is important to take the full course of therapy to prevent a reoccurrence of the infection.

| Generic Name<br>*Brand Name* | Side Effects | Warnings | Dosing | Notes |
|---|---|---|---|---|
| **Lincomycin**<br>*Lincocin* capsule<br>(℞) | Nausea, vomiting, diarrhea, bloody stools, flaking skin, vaginal infection, sore throat, unpleasant taste. | Notify a doctor if severe diarrhea, bloody stools, or unusual bleeding occurs. | May take without regard to food. | Used to treat topical acne. |
| **Methenamine Hippurate**<br>*Hiprex, Urex* tablet<br>(℞) | Bladder irritation, painful urination, nausea, diarrhea, edema. | Avoid citrus fruit, milk products, and medications with bicarbonate that can decrease the acidity of the urine. | May cause stomach upset so take with food. Vitamin C may increase its effectiveness. | Used to suppress or eliminate bacteria in the urine that cause urinary tract infections. |
| **Methenamine Mandelate**<br>*Mandelamine* tablet, suspension (℞) | Bladder irritation, painful urination, nausea, diarrhea, edema. | Avoid citrus fruit, milk products, and medications with bicarbonate that can decrease the acidity of the urine. | May cause stomach upset so take with food. Vitamin C may increase its effectiveness. | Used to suppress or eliminate bacteria in the urine that cause urinary tract infections. |
| **Metronidazole**<br>*Flagyl, Protostat* tablet (℞) | Nausea, vomiting, diarrhea, stomachache, vertigo, depression, flushing, dry mouth, nasal congestion. | Avoid alcoholic beverages and products containing alcohol during therapy and for at least 1 day after therapy is stopped. | May cause stomach upset so take with food. | Used for numerous infections. May cause urine to darken, which is not a cause for alarm. |

**ACTION** Antibiotics kill bacteria by preventing the formation of the normal cell bacterial wall increasing the likelihood that the cell will rupture. Allergic reactions include mild itching, rash, fever, joint pain, chest tightness, difficult breathing, and chills, and should be reported to your physician.

**INDICATION** Used to treat infections caused by bacteria. It is important to take the full course of therapy to prevent a reoccurrence of the infection.

| Generic Name<br>Brand Name | Side Effects | Warnings | Dosing | Notes |
|---|---|---|---|---|
| **Nalidixic Acid**<br>*NegGram* tablet,<br>suspension (℞) | Nausea, diarrhea, weakness, dizziness, joint pain, visual disturbances. | May cause drowsiness. Caution should be used with tasks requiring alertness. May increase sensitivity to sunlight. | May cause stomach upset so take with food. | Used to treat urinary tract infections. |
| **Neomycin Sulfate**<br>*Mycifradin* tablet (℞) | Nausea, vomiting, diarrhea, dizziness. | Notify a doctor if ringing in the ears or problems urinating develop. | Drink plenty of fluids. | Used to treat hepatic coma. |
| **Nitrofurantoin**<br>*Macrobid,*<br>*Macrodantin*<br>capsule (℞)<br>*Furadantin* suspension (℞) | Nausea, stomachache, dizziness, vertigo, weakness, joint pain, vision problems. | Brownish discoloration of urine may occur and is normal. | May cause stomach upset so take with food. Avoid antacids containing magnesium. | Used to treat urinary tract infections. |
| **Trimethoprim**<br>*Proloprim,*<br>*Trimpex* tablet (℞) | Stomach upset, nausea, vomiting, peeling skin, fever, anemia. | | Drink plenty of fluids. | Used to treat urinary tract infections. |
| **Vancomycin HCl**<br>*Vancocin* capsule,<br>solution (℞) | Nausea, chills, rash, fever, difficult breathing. | Notify a doctor if severe diarrhea, bloody stools, or unusual bleeding occurs. | | Store solution in the refrigerator. |

# Antifungals

**ACTION** Antifungals typically interfere with the formation of the fungi's cell membrane. This results in leakage of cellular contents and death of the fungi cells.

**INDICATION** Used to treat various fungal infections such as athlete's foot, jock itch, ringworm, Tinea versicolor, candidiasis (yeast), and eczema. It is important to take or use the full course of therapy to prevent a recurrence of the infection.

| Generic Name<br>*Brand Name* | Side Effects | Warnings | Dosing | Notes |
|---|---|---|---|---|
| **Clotrimazole**<br>*Mycelex* troche (℞) | Nausea, vomiting. | | Dissolve slowly in mouth. | Troche used to treat oral thrush. |
| **Fluconazole**<br>*Diflucan* tablet, suspension (℞) | Nausea, vomiting, diarrhea, indigestion, headache, rash, dizziness. | | | Used to treat yeast infections of the mouth, throat, and vagina, and other Candida infections. |
| **Flucytosine**<br>*5-FC, Ancobon* capsule (℞) | Nausea, vomiting, diarrhea, indigestion, headache, rash, dizziness. | | Make cause stomach upset so take with food. | |
| **Griseofulvin**<br>*Grisactin, Fulvicin, Gris-Peg* tablet, capsule, suspension (℞) | Nausea, diarrhea, stomachache, headache, fatigue. Confusion, sleeplessness, hives. | May cause sensitivity to sunlight. | Take with food high in fat content. | Used to treat ringworm infections of the hair, skin, and nails, and for treatment of athlete's foot. |
| **Itraconazole**<br>*Sporanox* capsule, solution (℞) | GI upset, diarrhea, nausea, vomiting, stomach pain, headache, dizziness, fatigue, fever, muscle pain. | Birth control recommended during therapy and for 2 months after. | Take after a full meal. | Used for fungal infections such as histoplasmosis. |
| **Ketoconazole**<br>*Nizoral* tablet (℞) | Tablets may cause nausea, stomachache. | | Take tablets with food to avoid stomach upset. | Tablet used for internal fungal infections. |

Anti-Infectives

**ACTION** Antifungals typically interfere with the formation of the fungi's cell membrane. This results in leakage of cellular contents and death of the fungi cells.

**INDICATION** Used to treat various fungal infections such as athlete's foot, jock itch, ringworm, Tinea versicolor, candidiasis (yeast), and eczema. It is important to take or use the full course of therapy to prevent a recurrence of the infection.

| Generic Name<br>Brand Name | Side Effects | Warnings | Dosing | Notes |
|---|---|---|---|---|
| **Nystatin**<br>*Nilstat, Mycostatin*<br>tablet, suspension (℞) | Nausea, vomiting, diarrhea, stomachache, swelling, dryness. | | Suspension should be shaken well. | To treat oral, intestinal, or skin infections of Candida (yeast). |

## Antimalarials

**ACTION** Most antimalarial drugs interfere with DNA or RNA of malaria-causing organisms.

**INDICATION** Used to prevent and/or treat attacks of malaria.

| Generic Name<br>Brand Name | Side Effects | Warnings | Dosing | Notes |
|---|---|---|---|---|
| **Chloroquine Phosphate**<br>*Aralen* tablet (℞) | Nausea, vomiting, diarrhea, low blood pressure, pigment changes, tinnitus, headache. | Notify a doctor if stomach pain, diarrhea, muscle weakness, or vomiting occurs. Report any vision changes. | May cause stomach upset so take with food. | Used as an amebicide. If used long-term, periodic eye exams should occur. |
| **Hydroxychloroquine Sulfate**<br>*Plaquenil* tablet (℞) | Nausea, vomiting, diarrhea, low blood pressure, pigment changes, ringing in the ears, headache. | Notify a doctor if stomach pain, diarrhea, muscle weakness, or vomiting occurs. Report any vision changes. | May cause stomach upset so take with food. | Used to treat rheumatoid arthritis and lupus. If used long-term, periodic eye exams should occur. |
| **Mefloquine HCl**<br>*Lariam* tablet (℞) | Nausea, vomiting, diarrhea, vertigo, headache, ringing in the ears, chills, fever, fatigue. | Notify a doctor if anxiety, depression, restlessness, or confusion develops. | Do not take on an empty stomach. | |

**ACTION** Most antimalarial drugs interfere with DNA or RNA of malaria-causing organisms.

**INDICATION** Used to prevent and/or treat attacks of malaria.

| Generic Name<br>*Brand Name* | Side Effects | Warnings | Dosing | Notes |
|---|---|---|---|---|
| **Primaquine Phosphate**<br>*Primaquine* tablet (℞) | Nausea, vomiting, diarrhea, low blood pressure, pigment changes, ringing in the ears, headache. | Notify a doctor if stomach pain, diarrhea, muscle weakness, or vomiting occurs. Report any vision changes. | May cause stomach upset so take with food. | If used long-term, periodic eye exams should occur. |
| **Pyrimethamine**<br>*Daraprim* tablet (℞) | Nausea, vomiting, diarrhea, insomnia, headache. | Notify a doctor if stomach pain, diarrhea, muscle weakness, or vomiting occurs. | May cause stomach upset so take with food. | |
| **Quinine Sulfate**<br>*Quinamm* tablet (℞) | Nausea, vomiting, low blood pressure, chest pain, ringing in the ears, headache, night blindness, blurred vision, flushing. | Notify a doctor if stomach pain, diarrhea, muscle weakness, or vomiting occurs. | May cause stomach upset so take with food. | |

Anti-Infectives

# Antituberculous

**ACTION** These medications are either bactericidal (destructive to mycobacteria) or bacteriostatic (inhibit the growth of mycobacteria). They are commonly used in combination with each other.

**INDICATION** These medications either are used for treatment of tuberculous or for retreatment.

| Generic Name Brand Name | Side Effects | Warnings | Dosing | Notes |
|---|---|---|---|---|
| **Cycloserine** *Seromycin* capsule (℞) | Nausea, diarrhea, dizziness, confusion, weakness, slurred speech, tremor, anemia. | May cause drowsiness. Use caution when performing tasks that require alertness. | | Bacteriostatic. May be used to treat urinary tract infections. |
| **Ethambutol** *Myambutol* tablet (℞) | Nausea, diarrhea, dizziness, confusion, weakness, disorientation, gout, joint pain. | | Take with food to avoid stomach upset. | Bacteriostatic. |
| **Ethionamide** *Trecator-SC* tablet (℞) | Nausea, diarrhea, dizziness, confusion, weakness, salivation, tremors, depression. | | Take with food to avoid upset stomach, metallic taste, or appetite loss. | Bacteriostatic. |
| **Isoniazid** *Laniazid* tablet (℞) | Nausea, diarrhea, dizziness, confusion, weakness, increased blood sugar, niacin deficiency. | Minimize alcohol use. | Take on an empty stomach. | Bactericidal. |
| **Isoniazid, Rifampin** *Rifamate* capsule (℞) | Nausea, diarrhea, dizziness, confusion, weakness, increased blood sugar, niacin deficiency, cramps, flushing. | Minimize alcohol use. | Take on an empty stomach. | Bactericidal. May discolor urine, which is not harmful. |
| **Pyrazinamide** tablet (℞) | Nausea, diarrhea, anemia, rash. | May increase sensitivity to sunlight. | | Bacteriostatic. |

**ACTION** These medications are either bactericidal (destructive to mycobacteria) or bacteriostatic (inhibit the growth of mycobacteria). They are commonly used in combination with each other.

**INDICATION** These medications either are used for treatment of tuberculous or for retreatment.

| Generic Name Brand Name | Side Effects | Warnings | Dosing | Notes |
|---|---|---|---|---|
| **Rifabutin** *Mycobutin* capsule (℞) | Nausea, diarrhea, dizziness, confusion, weakness, chest pain, indigestion. | Minimize alcohol use. | Take on an empty stomach. | Bacteriostatic. May discolor urine, which is not harmful. |
| **Rifampin** *Rifadin* capsule (℞) | Nausea, diarrhea, dizziness, confusion, weakness, cramps, flushing. | | Take on an empty stomach. | Bactericidal. May discolor urine, which is not harmful. |

## Antiviral—Protease Inhibitors

**ACTION** Inhibit the viral proteases of HIV, resulting in the inhibition of viral replication. They do not eliminate the virus and are not a cure, nor do they prevent transmission of the virus.

**INDICATION** Used for the treatment of patients infected with the HIV virus in combination with other antiviral medications. More than one protease inhibitor may be used concurrently. It is important that the therapy not be interrupted.

| Generic Name Brand Name | Side Effects | Warnings | Dosing | Notes |
|---|---|---|---|---|
| **Indinavir Sulfate** *Crixivan* (℞) | Chest pain, chills, flulike symptoms, malaise, pain, syncope. | | Take 1 hour before or 2 hours after food and with a full glass of water. | |
| **Ritonavir** *Norvir* capsule (℞) | Nausea, diarrhea, vomiting, constipation, weakness, numbness, dizziness. | | Take with food or milk. | Store in refrigerator. |

**ACTION** Inhibit the viral proteases of HIV, resulting in the inhibition of viral replication. They do not eliminate the virus and are not a cure, nor do they prevent transmission of the virus.

**INDICATION** Used for the treatment of patients infected with the HIV virus in combination with other antiviral medications. More than one protease inhibitor may be used concurrently. It is important that the therapy not be interrupted.

| Generic Name<br>*Brand Name* | Side Effects | Warnings | Dosing | Notes |
|---|---|---|---|---|
| **Saquinavir Mesylate**<br>*Invirase* capsule (Ŗ) | Diarrhea, stomach pain, numbness, headache, muscle pain. | May cause sensitivity to sunlight. | Do not take with food or sooner than 2 hours after a full meal. | |

## Antiviral—Miscellaneous

**ACTION** Most antiviral medications work to inhibit the virus from reproducing or growing. They do not eliminate the virus and are not a cure, nor do they prevent transmission of the virus.

**INDICATION** Used for the treatment or prevention of various virus infections. It is important to take the full course of therapy as prescribed.

| Generic Name<br>*Brand Name* | Side Effects | Warnings | Dosing | Notes |
|---|---|---|---|---|
| **Acyclovir**<br>*Zovirax* capsule, tablet, suspension (Ŗ) | Nausea, vomiting, headache, rash, weakness. | Avoid sexual intercourse when sores are present to prevent infecting your partner. | | Used to treat shingles, genital herpes, chickenpox, and other herpes simplex infections of the body. |
| **Amantadine**<br>*Symmetrel, Symadine* capsule, syrup (Ŗ) | Nausea, dizziness, insomnia, depression, anxiety, orthostatic hypotension. | | | Used to prevent and treat influenza A virus infections, and to treat Parkinson's disease. |
| **Delaviridine Mesylate**<br>*Rescriptor* tablet (Ŗ) | Rash. | Avoid antacids within 2 hours before or after taking this drug. | May take without regard to meals. | |

**ACTION** Most antiviral medications work to inhibit the virus from reproducing or growing. They do not eliminate the virus and are not a cure, nor do they prevent transmission of the virus.

**INDICATION** Used for the treatment or prevention of various virus infections. It is important to take the full course of therapy as prescribed.

| Generic Name Brand Name | Side Effects | Warnings | Dosing | Notes |
|---|---|---|---|---|
| **Didanosine** ddl, Videx tablet, solution (℞) | Nausea, vomiting, diarrhea, headache, weakness, edema, muscle pain, appetite loss, confusion, high blood pressure. | Alcohol may increase the side effects. | Take on an empty stomach. | Used for the treatment of advanced HIV infection when zidovudine (AZT) can no longer be used. |
| **Famciclovir** Famvir tablet (℞) | Nausea, diarrhea, vomiting, constipation, headache, dizziness, fatigue, sore throat, sinus congestion, fever, pain. | Avoid sexual intercourse when sores are present to prevent infecting sex partner. | May take with food if stomach upset occurs. | Used to treat shingles and genital herpes. |
| **Ganciclovir Sodium** DHPG, Cytovene capsule (℞) | Nausea, vomiting, headache, weakness, infections, fever, vision changes. | | Take with food. Drink plenty of fluids. | For the treatment of cytomegalovirus (CMV). |
| **Lamivudine** 3TC, Epivir tablet (℞) | Nausea, diarrhea, numbness, sleep disorders, depression, fatigue. | | May be taken with or without food. | Used to treat HIV virus. |
| **Nelfinavir Mesylate** Viracept tablet, powder (℞) | Diarrhea, nausea, flatulence, rash. | | Take with a meal or light snack for optimal absorption. | |
| **Nevirapine** Viramune tablet (℞) | Rash, fever, nausea, headache. | | May take with or without food. | Used to treat HIV virus. |

Anti-Infectives

**ACTION** Most antiviral medications work to inhibit the virus from reproducing or growing. They do not eliminate the virus and are not a cure, nor do they prevent transmission of the virus.

**INDICATION** Used for the treatment or prevention of various virus infections. It is important to take the full course of therapy as prescribed.

| Generic Name Brand Name | Side Effects | Warnings | Dosing | Notes |
|---|---|---|---|---|
| **Rimantadine** *Flumadine* tablet, syrup (℞) | Nausea, vomiting, stomach pain, dry mouth, tiredness, weakness, insomnia. | May cause drowsiness. Use caution when performing tasks that require alertness. | | Used to prevent and treat influenza A virus. |
| **Stavudine** *d4T, Zerit* capsule (℞) | Headache, muscle pain, diarrhea, nausea, vomiting, constipation. | | May take with or without food. | Used for treatment of HIV virus. |
| **Valacyclovir** *Valtrex* caplet (℞) | Nausea, vomiting, diarrhea, constipation, headache, abdominal pain, anorexia. | Avoid sexual intercourse when sores are present to prevent infecting sex partner. | May take without regard to food. | Used to treat shingles. |
| **Zalcitabine** *ddC, Hivid* tablet (℞) | Nausea, appetite loss, stomach pain, dizziness, chest pain, high blood pressure. | May cause sensitivity to sunlight. May affect blood sugar of diabetics. | Do not take at the same time as antacids. | Used to inhibit the growth of the HIV virus. |
| **Zidovudine** *AZT, Retrovir* capsule, syrup (℞) | Appetite loss, nausea, vomiting, weakness, dizziness, drowsiness, anemia. | | Take exactly as prescribed. | |

# Central Nervous System Agents

## Antianxiety

**ACTION** Antianxiety drugs reduce anxiety by affecting chemicals in the brain.

**INDICATION** Used to treat anxiety disorders and for short-term relief of symptoms of anxiety. Some of these substances can be addictive.

| Generic Name<br>*Brand Name* | Side Effects | Warnings | Dosing | Notes |
|---|---|---|---|---|
| **Alprazolam**<br>*Xanax* tablet<br>(℞, C-IV) | Stomach upset, constipation, diarrhea, confusion, depression, behavior changes, fatigue, changes in blood pressure, incontinence, vision disturbances. | Use caution when performing tasks requiring alertness. Avoid alcohol and other drugs causing drowsiness. | | Also indicated for the treatment of panic disorder, with or without agoraphobia, and for treatment of anxiety associated with depression. |
| **Buspirone**<br>*BuSpar* tablet (℞) | Dizziness, nausea, headache, nervousness, lightheadedness, excitement. | Use caution when performing tasks requiring alertness. Avoid alcohol and other drugs that cause drowsiness. | | |
| **Chlordiazepoxide**<br>*Librium* capsule<br>(℞, C-IV) | Stomach upset, constipation, diarrhea, confusion, depression, behavior changes, fatigue, changes in blood pressure, incontinence, vision disturbances. | Use caution when performing tasks requiring alertness. Avoid alcohol and other drugs that cause drowsiness. | | Also used for the treatment of alcohol withdrawal symptoms. |

**ACTION** Antianxiety drugs reduce anxiety by affecting chemicals in the brain.

**INDICATION** Used to treat anxiety disorders and for short-term relief of symptoms of anxiety. Some of these substances can be addictive.

| Generic Name<br>*Brand Name* | Side Effects | Warnings | Dosing | Notes |
|---|---|---|---|---|
| **Clonazepam**<br>*Klonopin* tablet<br>(℞, C-IV) | Stomach upset, constipation, diarrhea, confusion, depression, behavior changes, fatigue, changes in blood pressure, incontinence, vision disturbances. | Use caution when performing tasks requiring alertness. Avoid alcohol and other drugs that cause drowsiness. | Use of antacids may impair absorption. | Used in the management of seizures in combination with other drugs. |
| **Clorazepate Dipotassium**<br>*Tranxene* tablet, capsule (℞, C-IV) | Stomach upset, constipation, diarrhea, confusion, depression, behavior changes, fatigue, changes in blood pressure, incontinence, vision disturbances. | Use caution when performing tasks requiring alertness. Avoid alcohol and other drugs that cause drowsiness. | Use of antacids may impair absorption. | Used in treatment of symptoms of alcohol withdrawal and for management of seizures in combination with other drugs. |
| **Diazepam**<br>*Valium, Valrelease* tablet, capsule (℞, C-IV) | Stomach upset, constipation, diarrhea, confusion, depression, behavior changes, fatigue, changes in blood pressure, incontinence, vision disturbances. | Use caution when performing tasks requiring alertness. Avoid alcohol and other drugs that cause drowsiness. | Use of antacids may impair absorption. | Used in treatment of acute agitation, muscle spasms, and in combination with other drugs to control convulsions. |
| **Halazepam**<br>*Paxipam* tablet<br>(℞, C-IV) | Stomach upset, constipation, diarrhea, confusion, depression, behavior changes, fatigue, changes in blood pressure, incontinence, vision disturbances. | Use caution when performing tasks requiring alertness. Avoid alcohol and other drugs that cause drowsiness. | | |

**ACTION** Antianxiety drugs reduce anxiety by affecting chemicals in the brain.

**INDICATION** Used to treat anxiety disorders and for short-term relief of symptoms of anxiety. Some of these substances can be addictive.

| Generic Name<br>*Brand Name* | Side Effects | Warnings | Dosing | Notes |
|---|---|---|---|---|
| **Hydroxyzine HCl**<br>*Atarax* tablet (℞) | Tremor, seizures, dizziness, dry mouth, involuntary movements. | Use caution when performing tasks requiring alertness. Avoid alcohol and other drugs that cause drowsiness. | | Also used for treatment of itching from rash, hives, and insect bites. |
| **Hydroxyzine Pamoate**<br>*Vistaril* capsule (℞) | Tremor, seizures, dizziness, dry mouth, involuntary movements. | Use caution when performing tasks requiring alertness. Avoid alcohol and other drugs that cause drowsiness. | | Also used for treatment of itching from rash, hives, and insect bites. |
| **Lorazepam**<br>*Ativan* tablet<br>(℞, C-IV) | Stomach upset, constipation, diarrhea, confusion, depression, behavior changes, fatigue, changes in blood pressure, incontinence, vision disturbances. | Use caution when performing tasks requiring alertness. Avoid alcohol and other drugs that cause drowsiness. | | Also used for the treatment of anxiety associated with depression. |
| **Meprobamate**<br>*Equanil, Miltown* tablet (℞, C-IV) | Stomach upset, nausea, vomiting, diarrhea, dizziness, vertigo, overstimulation, chills, low blood pressure. | Use caution when performing tasks requiring alertness. Avoid alcohol and other drugs that cause drowsiness. | | |

**ACTION** Antianxiety drugs reduce anxiety by affecting chemicals in the brain.

**INDICATION** Used to treat anxiety disorders and for short-term relief of symptoms of anxiety. Some of these substances can be addictive.

| Generic Name<br>*Brand Name* | Side Effects | Warnings | Dosing | Notes |
|---|---|---|---|---|
| **Oxazepam**<br>*Serax* capsule<br>(℞, C-IV) | Stomach upset, constipation, diarrhea, confusion, depression, behavior changes, fatigue, changes in blood pressure, incontinence, vision disturbances. | Use caution when performing tasks requiring alertness. Avoid alcohol and other drugs that cause drowsiness. | | Used in the treatment of anxiety associated with depression or alcohol withdrawal. |
| **Prazepam**<br>*Centrax* tablet, capsule (℞, C-IV) | Stomach upset, constipation, diarrhea, confusion, depression, behavior changes, fatigue, changes in blood pressure, incontinence, vision disturbances. | Use caution when performing tasks requiring alertness. Avoid alcohol and other drugs that cause drowsiness. | | |

## Anticonvulsants

**ACTION** These medications prevent or reduce seizures by decreasing the activity of nerve impulses in the brain and central nervous system. Some sedative-barbiturates may also be used as anticonvulsants.

**INDICATION** Used to treat seizures associated with disorders such as epilepsy, petit mal, grand mal, and other psychomotor seizures.

| Generic Name<br>*Brand Name* | Side Effects | Warnings | Dosing | Notes |
|---|---|---|---|---|
| **Carbamazepine**<br>*Epitol, Tegretol* tablet, suspension (℞) | Nausea, vomiting, dizziness, blood pressure changes, fatigue, blurred vision. | May cause drowsiness. Use caution when performing tasks that require alertness. | Take with food to avoid stomach upset. | Also used to treat trigeminal neuralgia. |

**ACTION** These medications prevent or reduce seizures by decreasing the activity of nerve impulses in the brain and central nervous system. Some sedative-barbiturates may also be used as anticonvulsants.

**INDICATION** Used to treat seizures associated with disorders such as epilepsy, petit mal, grand mal, and other psychomotor seizures.

| Generic Name<br>*Brand Name* | Side Effects | Warnings | Dosing | Notes |
|---|---|---|---|---|
| **Clonazepam**<br>*Klonopin* tablet<br>(℞, C-IV) | Constipation, nausea, confusion, depression, tremor, vertigo, difficult breathing, blurred vision. | May cause drowsiness. Use caution when performing tasks that require alertness. Alcohol and other depressants can intensify side effects. | Take with food to avoid stomach upset. | May also be prescribed for panic attacks. |
| **Ethosuximide**<br>*Zarontin* capsule, syrup (℞) | Nausea, vomiting, appetite loss, dizziness, nervousness, hyperactivity, depression. | May cause drowsiness. Use caution when performing tasks that require alertness. Alcohol and other depressants may intensify this effect. | Take with food to avoid stomach upset. | |
| **Felbamate**<br>*Felbatol* tablet (℞) | Vomiting, constipation, appetite loss, sleeplessness, anxiety, stupor, anemia. | May cause sensitivity to sunlight or sun lamps. | May be taken with or without food. | |
| **Gabapentin**<br>*Neurontin* capsule (℞) | Appetite changes, indigestion, hyperactivity, drowsiness, anxiety, incoordination, fatigue. | May cause drowsiness. Use caution when performing tasks that require alertness. | Wait at least 2 hours after antacids before taking. | |

**ACTION** These medications prevent or reduce seizures by decreasing the activity of nerve impulses in the brain and central nervous system. Some sedative-barbiturates may also be used as anticonvulsants.

**INDICATION** Used to treat seizures associated with disorders such as epilepsy, petit mal, grand mal, and other psychomotor seizures.

| Generic Name<br>*Brand Name* | Side Effects | Warnings | Dosing | Notes |
|---|---|---|---|---|
| **Lamotrigine**<br>*Lamictal* tablet (℞) | Stomachache, nausea, appetite loss, dizziness, incoordination, hot flashes, headache. | May cause drowsiness. Use caution when performing tasks that require alertness. May cause sensitivity to sunlight. | May be taken without regard to food. | |
| **Mephenytoin**<br>*Mesantoin* tablet (℞) | Nausea, persistent headache, tremor, dizziness, nervousness, joint pain, confusion. | Avoid alcoholic beverages. | Take with food to avoid stomach upset. | Maintain good oral hygiene. |
| **Methsuximide**<br>*Celontin* capsule (℞) | Nausea, vomiting, appetite loss, dizziness, nervousness, hyperactivity, depression. | May cause drowsiness. Use caution when performing tasks that require alertness. Alcohol and other depressants may intensify this effect. | Take with food to avoid stomach upset. | |
| **Phensuximide**<br>*Milontin* capsule (℞) | Nausea, vomiting, appetite loss, dizziness, nervousness, hyperactivity, depression. | May cause drowsiness. Use caution when performing tasks that require alertness. Alcohol and other depressants may intensify this effect. | Take with food to avoid stomach upset. | |

**ACTION** These medications prevent or reduce seizures by decreasing the activity of nerve impulses in the brain and central nervous system. Some sedative-barbiturates may also be used as anticonvulsants.

**INDICATION** Used to treat seizures associated with disorders such as epilepsy, petit mal, grand mal, and other psychomotor seizures.

| Generic Name<br>*Brand Name* | Side Effects | Warnings | Dosing | Notes |
|---|---|---|---|---|
| **Phenytoin**<br>*Dilantin* tablet, capsule, suspension (℞) | Nausea, persistent headache, tremor, dizziness, nervousness, joint pain, confusion. | Avoid alcoholic beverages. | Take with food to avoid stomach upset. | Maintain good oral hygiene. |
| **Primidone**<br>*Mysoline* tablet, suspension (℞) | Nausea, vomiting, clumsiness, tiredness, blurred vision. | May cause drowsiness. Use caution when performing tasks that require alertness. Alcohol and other depressants may intensify this effect. | Take with food to avoid stomach upset. | |
| **Topiramate**<br>*Topamax* tablet (℞) | Ataxia, dizziness, fatigue, nervousness, somnolence, weight loss. | May cause drowsiness. Use caution when performing tasks that require alertness. | May be taken with or without food. | |
| **Valproic Acid**<br>*Depakene* capsule, syrup (℞)<br>*Depakote* tablet (℞) | Vision changes, appetite changes, nausea, weakness, clumsiness, tremors, blood pressure changes, flushing. | May cause drowsiness. Use caution when performing tasks that require alertness. Alcohol and other depressants may intensify this effect. May cause sensitivity to sunlight. | Take with food to avoid stomach upset. | Used to treat manic episodes associated with bipolar disorders. |

Central Nervous System

## Antidepressants—MAOIs

**ACTION** Monoamine oxidase inhibitors (MAOIs) inhibit a complex enzyme system, thus increasing epinephrine, serotonin, and norepinephrine in the brain. An antidepressant's effect may take a few weeks to be noticed. Do not stop therapy unless instructed by a doctor.

**INDICATION** Used to treat atypical depression, bulimia, panic disorders, and depression not responsive to other therapies. These medications interact with numerous medications and any foods containing tyramine.

| Generic Name<br>Brand Name | Side Effects | Warnings | Dosing | Notes |
|---|---|---|---|---|
| **Isocarboxazid**<br>*Marplan* tablet (℞) | Nausea, constipation, hyperactivity, tremors, excitement, irritability, orthostatic hypotension, flushing, weight changes, edema. | May cause drowsiness. Use caution when performing tasks that require alertness. | Avoid tyramine-containing foods, alcohol, and caffeine. | |
| **Phenelzine**<br>*Nardil* tablet (℞) | Nausea, constipation, hyperactivity, tremors, excitement, irritability, orthostatic hypotension, flushing, weight changes, edema. | May cause drowsiness. Use caution when performing tasks that require alertness. | Avoid tyramine-containing foods, alcohol, and caffeine. | |
| **Tranylcypromine**<br>*Parnate* tablet (℞) | Nausea, constipation, hyperactivity, tremors, excitement, irritability, orthostatic hypotension, flushing, weight changes, edema. | May cause drowsiness. Use caution when performing tasks that require alertness. | Avoid tyramine-containing foods, alcohol, and caffeine. | |

# Antidepressants—SSRIs

**ACTION** Selective serotonin reuptake inhibitors (SSRIs) work by a variety of known and unknown mechanisms. Chemicals in the brain affected include serotonin and norepinephrine. An antidepressant's effect may take a few weeks to be noticed. Do not stop therapy unless instructed by a doctor.

**INDICATION** Used to treat mental depression.

| Generic Name<br>*Brand Name* | Side Effects | Warnings | Dosing | Notes |
|---|---|---|---|---|
| **Fluoxetine HCl**<br>*Prozac* capsule (℞) | Stomach upset, indigestion, tremors, anxiety, flulike syndrome, sweating, chest pain, edema. | Use caution when performing tasks requiring alertness or physical dexterity. Diabetics may experience hypoglycemia. | Avoid alcohol and other depressants that increase drowsiness. Take in the morning to avoid insomnia. | Used for Obsessive Compulsive Disorder (OCD), bulimia, and other mental and physical disorders. |
| **Fluvoxamine Maleate**<br>*Luvox* tablet (℞) | Nausea, vomiting, memory loss, indifference, incoordination, chest pain, rapid heart beat, sweating. | Use caution when performing tasks requiring alertness or physical dexterity. | Avoid alcohol and smoking. | Used for Obsessive Compulsive Disorder (OCD). |
| **Paroxetine**<br>*Paxil* tablet (℞) | Nausea, diarrhea, constipation, sleeplessness, agitation, anxiety, chest pain, flushing, weight loss. | May cause drowsiness. Use caution when performing tasks that require alertness. | | |
| **Sertraline**<br>*Zoloft* tablet (℞) | Nausea, diarrhea, constipation, sleeplessness, agitation, anxiety, chest pain, flushing, weight loss. | May cause drowsiness. Use caution when performing tasks that require alertness. | | |

**ACTION** Selective serotonin reuptake inhibitors (SSRIs) work by a variety of known and unknown mechanisms. Chemicals in the brain affected include serotonin and norepinephrine. An antidepressant's effect may take a few weeks to be noticed. Do not stop therapy unless instructed by a doctor.

**INDICATION** Used to treat mental depression.

| Generic Name<br>*Brand Name* | Side Effects | Warnings | Dosing | Notes |
|---|---|---|---|---|
| **Venlafaxine HCl**<br>*Effexor* tablet (℞),<br>*Effexor XR* extended release<br>capsule (℞) | Nausea, diarrhea, constipation, sleeplessness, agitation, anxiety, chest pain, flushing, weight loss. | May cause drowsiness. Use caution when performing tasks that require alertness. | | |

## Antidepressants—TCAs

**ACTION** Tricyclic antidepressants (TCAs) inhibit the reuptake of norepinephrine and serotonin at the presynaptic neuron. The TCAs' effect may take a few weeks to be noticed. Do not stop therapy unless instructed by a doctor. Avoid sunlight and sun lamps as TCAs may cause photosensitivity.

**INDICATION** Used to relieve symptoms of depression. TCAs with significant sedative action may also be used for depression associated with anxiety and sleep disturbances.

| Generic Name<br>*Brand Name* | Side Effects | Warnings | Dosing | Notes |
|---|---|---|---|---|
| **Amitriptyline HCl**<br>*Elavil, Endep* tablet<br>(℞) | Nausea, constipation, anxiety, excitement, disturbed concentration, rapid pulse, chest pain, photosensitivity. | May cause drowsiness. Use caution when performing tasks that require alertness. Use with alcohol may intensify these effects. | Taking drug at bedtime may reduce some side effects. | May also be used for bulimia, chronic pain, cluster headaches, and migraine headaches. |

**ACTION** Tricyclic antidepressants (TCAs) inhibit the reuptake of norepinephrine and serotonin at the presynaptic neuron. The TCAs' effect may take a few weeks to be noticed. Do not stop therapy unless instructed by a doctor. Avoid sunlight and sun lamps as TCAs may cause photosensitivity.

**INDICATION** Used to relieve symptoms of depression. TCAs with significant sedative action may also be used for depression associated with anxiety and sleep disturbances.

| Generic Name Brand Name | Side Effects | Warnings | Dosing | Notes |
|---|---|---|---|---|
| **Amitriptyline HCl, Chlordiazep- oxide** *Limbitrol* tablet (℞, C-IV) | Nausea, consti- pation, anxiety, excitement, dis- turbed concen- tration, rapid pulse, chest pain, photosensitivity. | May cause drowsiness. Use caution when performing tasks that re- quire alertness. Use with alcohol may intensify these effects. | Taking drug at bedtime may re- duce some side effects. | May also be used for bulimia, chronic pain, cluster head- aches, and migraine headaches. |
| **Amitriptyline HCl, Perphenazine** *Etrafon, Triavil* (℞) | Nausea, consti- pation, anxiety, excitement, dis- turbed concen- tration, rapid pulse, chest pain, photosensitivity. | May cause drowsiness. Use caution when perform- ing tasks that re- quire alertness. Use with alcohol may intensify these effects. | Taking drug at bedtime may re- duce some side effects. | May also be used for bulimia, chronic pain, cluster head- aches, and migraine headaches. |
| **Amoxapine** *Asendin* tablet (℞) | Nausea, consti- pation, anxiety, excitement, dis- turbed concen- tration, rapid pulse, chest pain, sensitivity to light. | May cause drowsiness. Use caution when performing tasks that require alertness. Use with alcohol may intensify these effects. | Taking drug at bedtime may re- duce some side effects. | |
| **Clomipramine HCl** *Anafranil* capsule (℞) | Nausea, consti- pation, anxiety, excitement, dis- turbed concen- tration, rapid pulse, chest pain, sensitivity to light. | May cause drowsiness. Use caution when performing tasks that require alertness. Use with alcohol may intensify these effects. | Taking drug at bedtime may re- duce some side effects. | Only used for treatment of Obsessive Com- pulsive Disorder (OCD). |

**ACTION** Tricyclic antidepressants (TCAs) inhibit the reuptake of norepinephrine and serotonin at the presynaptic neuron. The TCAs' effect may take a few weeks to be noticed. Do not stop therapy unless instructed by a doctor. Avoid sunlight and sun lamps as TCAs may cause photosensitivity.

**INDICATION** Used to relieve symptoms of depression. TCAs with significant sedative action may also be used for depression associated with anxiety and sleep disturbances.

| Generic Name<br>*Brand Name* | Side Effects | Warnings | Dosing | Notes |
|---|---|---|---|---|
| **Desipramine HCl**<br>*Norpramin* tablet (℞)<br>*Pertofrane* capsule (℞) | Nausea, constipation, anxiety, excitement, disturbed concentration, rapid pulse, chest pain, sensitivity to light. | May cause drowsiness. Use caution when performing tasks that require alertness. Use with alcohol may intensify these effects. | Taking drug at bedtime may reduce some side effects. | May also be used for bulimia, chronic pain, cluster head aches, and migraine headaches. |
| **Imipramine**<br>*Tofranil* tablet (℞)<br>*Tofranil-PM* capsule (℞) | Nausea, constipation, anxiety, excitement, disturbed concentration, rapid pulse, chest pain, sensitivity to light. | May cause drowsiness. Use caution when performing tasks that require alertness. Use with alcohol may intensify these effects. | Taking drug at bedtime may reduce some side effects. | Used in the treatment of bed-wetting in children and panic disorder in adults. |
| **Nortriptyline HCl**<br>*Aventyl, Pamelor* capsule, solution (℞) | Nausea, constipation, anxiety, excitement, disturbed concentration, rapid pulse, chest pain, sensitivity to light. | May cause drowsiness. Use caution when performing tasks that require alertness. Use with alcohol may intensify these effects. | Taking drug at bedtime may reduce some side effects. | May also be used for premenstrual depression. |
| **Protriptyline HCl**<br>*Vivactil* tablet (℞) | Nausea, constipation, anxiety, excitement, disturbed concentration, rapid pulse, chest pain, sensitivity to light. | May cause drowsiness. Use caution when performing tasks that require alertness. Use with alcohol may intensify these effects. | Taking drug at bedtime may reduce some side effects. | May also be used for obstructive sleep apnea. |

**ACTION** Tricyclic antidepressants (TCAs) inhibit the reuptake of norepinephrine and serotonin at the presynaptic neuron. The TCAs' effect may take a few weeks to be noticed. Do not stop therapy unless instructed by a doctor. Avoid sunlight and sun lamps as TCAs may cause photosensitivity.

**INDICATION** Used to relieve symptoms of depression. TCAs with significant sedative action may also be used for depression associated with anxiety and sleep disturbances.

| Generic Name<br>*Brand Name* | Side Effects | Warnings | Dosing | Notes |
| --- | --- | --- | --- | --- |
| **Trimipramine<br>Maleate**<br>*Surmontil* capsule<br>(℞) | Nausea, constipation, anxiety, excitement, disturbed concentration, rapid pulse, chest pain, sensitivity to light. | May cause drowsiness. Use caution when performing tasks that require alertness. Use with alcohol may intensify these effects. | Taking drug at bedtime may reduce some side effects. | |

## Antidepressants—Miscellaneous

**ACTION** Antidepressants work by a variety of known and unknown mechanisms. Chemicals in the brain affected include serotonin and norepinephrine. An antidepressant's effect may take a few weeks to be noticed. Do not stop therapy unless instructed by a doctor.

**INDICATION** Used to treat mental depression.

| Generic Name<br>*Brand Name* | Side Effects | Warnings | Dosing | Notes |
| --- | --- | --- | --- | --- |
| **Bupropion HCl**<br>*Wellbutrin* tablet<br>(℞)<br>*Wellbutrin SR*<br>sustained-release tablet (℞) | Tremors, muscle stiffness, incoordination, seizures, nausea, vomiting, blood pressure changes. | May cause drowsiness. Use caution when performing tasks that require alertness or physical dexterity. Avoid alcohol and other depressants that increase drowsiness and risk of seizures. | | |

Central Nervous System

**ACTION** Antidepressants work by a variety of known and unknown mechanisms. Chemicals in the brain affected include serotonin and norepinephrine. An antidepressant's effect may take a few weeks to be noticed. Do not stop therapy unless instructed by a doctor.

**INDICATION** Used to treat mental depression.

| Generic Name<br>*Brand Name* | Side Effects | Warnings | Dosing | Notes |
|---|---|---|---|---|
| **Maprotiline HCl**<br>*Ludiomil* tablet (℞) | Nausea, constipation, confusion, seizures, rapid pulse, flushing. | Use caution when performing tasks requiring alertness or physical dexterity. Alcohol may increase drowsiness. | | Used for manic-depressive illness and anxiety associated with depression. |
| **Mirtazapine**<br>*Remeron* tablet (℞) | Sleepiness, dry mouth, increased appetite, weight gain, constipation, dizziness. | Use caution when performing tasks requiring alertness. | | |
| **Nefazodone HCl**<br>*Serzone* tablet (℞) | Nausea, constipation, dizziness, low blood pressure, chest pain, dry mouth. | Use caution when performing tasks requiring alertness or physical dexterity. Avoid alcohol. | Take on an empty stomach. | |
| **Trazodone**<br>*Desyrel* tablet (℞) | Nausea, diarrhea, constipation, sleeplessness, confusion, orthostatic hypotension, chest pain, blurred vision. | May cause drowsiness. Use caution when performing tasks that require alertness. Avoid alcohol. | Take with food. | Used for panic disorders or agoraphobia. |

## Antiemetics

**ACTION** These medications act in a variety of methods to reduce nausea, vomiting, motion sickness, and vertigo. Some antipsychotic-phenothiazine drugs are also used for nausea and vomiting.

**INDICATION** For nausea and vomiting depending on the cause. They may be used alone or in combination with other medications. Avoid alcohol and other CNS depressants that may intensify side effects.

| Generic Name<br>*Brand Name* | Side Effects | Warnings | Dosing | Notes |
|---|---|---|---|---|
| **Buclizine HCl**<br>*Bucladin-S* tablet<br>(℞) | Drowsiness, dry mouth, headache, jitteriness. | Use caution when performing tasks requiring alertness. | | Effective for motion sickness. |
| **Cyclizine**<br>*Marezine* tablet<br>(OTC) | Drowsiness, restlessness, excitation, dry mouth. | Use caution when performing tasks requiring alertness. | | Effective for motion sickness. |
| **Dimenhydrinate**<br>*Dramamine* tablet,<br>liquid (OTC) | Drowsiness, confusion, restlessness, excitation, dry mouth. | Use caution when performing tasks requiring alertness. | | Effective for motion sickness and vertigo. |
| **Diphenidol**<br>*Vontrol* tablet (℞) | Drowsiness, disorientation, confusion, headache, blurred vision. | Use caution when performing tasks requiring alertness. | | Effective for vertigo. |
| **Dronabinol**<br>*Marinol* capsule<br>(℞, C-II) | Drowsiness, euphoria, anxiety, dizziness, depression. | Use caution when performing tasks requiring alertness. | | Used for nausea associated with chemotherapy. |
| **Granisetron HCl**<br>*Kytril* tablet (℞) | Headache, abdominal pain, constipation. | | | Used for nausea associated with chemotherapy. |
| **Meclizine**<br>*Bonine* tablet (OTC)<br>*Antivert* tablet (℞) | Drowsiness, restlessness, excitation, dry mouth. | Use caution when performing tasks requiring alertness. | | Effective for motion sickness and vertigo. |
| **Metoclopramide**<br>*Reglan* tablet,<br>syrup (℞) | | | | Used for nausea associated with chemotherapy. |

Central Nervous System

**ACTION** These medications act in a variety of methods to reduce nausea, vomiting, motion sickness, and vertigo. Some antipsychotic-phenothiazine drugs are also used for nausea and vomiting.

**INDICATION** For nausea and vomiting depending on the cause. They may be used alone or in combination with other medications. Avoid alcohol and other CNS depressants that may intensify side effects.

| Generic Name<br>*Brand Name* | Side Effects | Warnings | Dosing | Notes |
|---|---|---|---|---|
| **Ondansetron HCl**<br>*Zofran* tablet (℞) | Headache, abdominal pain, constipation, fatigue, sedation. | | | Used for nausea associated with chemotherapy. |
| **Phosphorated Carbohydrate Solution**<br>*Emetrol, Nausetrol* solution (OTC) | Diarrhea, abdominal pain. | Do not take any fluids 15 minutes before or after dose. | Do not dilute. | |
| **Promethazine HCl**<br>*Phenergan* tablet, suppository, syrup (℞) | Drowsiness, restlessness, excitation, dry mouth. | Use caution when performing tasks requiring alertness. | | Drug is found in combination with numerous other products. |
| **Thiethylperazine Maleate**<br>*Torecan* tablet, suppository (℞) | Drowsiness, restlessness, excitation, dry mouth. | Use caution when performing tasks requiring alertness. | | |
| **Trimethobenzamide HCl**<br>*Tigan* capsule, suppository (℞) | Drowsiness, headache, diarrhea, muscle cramps, blurred vision. | Use caution when performing tasks requiring alertness. | | |

# Antiparkinson Agents

**ACTION** These medications reduce the frequency and severity of the symptoms of Parkinson's disease and drug-induced Parkinson-like symptoms. Symptoms include tremor, rigidity, posture disorders, and equilibrium disorders.

**INDICATION** Used alone or in combination with other medications for Parkinson's symptoms. These medications do not cure the cause of the symptom.

| Generic Name<br>*Brand Name* | Side Effects | Warnings | Dosing | Notes |
|---|---|---|---|---|
| **Amantadine**<br>*Symmetrel* capsule<br>(℞) | Nausea, diarrhea, constipation, twitching, mood swings, irregular heartbeat, flushing, increased sweating. | May cause drowsiness. Use caution when performing tasks that require alertness. May darken urine or sweat, which is not harmful. | To avoid stomach upset, take with food. | Used to treat influenza A virus. |
| **Benztropine Mesylate**<br>*Cogentin* tablet (℞) | Nausea, constipation, disorientation, memory loss, weakness, agitation, rapid heart rate, vision changes. | May cause drowsiness. Use caution when performing tasks that require alertness. | To avoid stomach upset, take with food. | |
| **Biperiden**<br>*Akineton* tablet (℞) | Nausea, constipation, disorientation, memory loss, weakness, agitation, rapid heart rate, vision changes. | May cause drowsiness. Use caution when performing tasks that require alertness. | To avoid stomach upset, take with food. | |
| **Bromocriptine Mesylate**<br>*Parlodel* tablet, capsule (℞) | Nausea, diarrhea, constipation, twitching, mood swings, irregular heartbeat, flushing, increased sweating. | May cause drowsiness. Use caution when performing tasks that require alertness. May darken urine or sweat, which is not harmful. | To avoid stomach upset, take with food. | |

Central Nervous System

**ACTION** These medications reduce the frequency and severity of the symptoms of Parkinson's disease and drug-induced Parkinson-like symptoms. Symptoms include tremor, rigidity, posture disorders, and equilibrium disorders.

**INDICATION** Used alone or in combination with other medications for Parkinson's symptoms. These medications do not cure the cause of the symptom.

| Generic Name<br>*Brand Name* | Side Effects | Warnings | Dosing | Notes |
|---|---|---|---|---|
| **Levodopa**<br>*Larodopa* tablet,<br>capsule (℞) | Nausea, diarrhea, constipation, twitching, mood swings, irregular heartbeat, flushing, increased sweating. | May cause drowsiness. Use caution when performing tasks that require alertness. May darken urine or sweat, which is not harmful. | To avoid stomach upset, take with food. | |
| **Levodopa,**<br>**Carbidopa**<br>*Sinemet* tablet (℞) | Nausea, diarrhea, constipation, twitching, mood swings, irregular heartbeat, flushing, increased sweating. | May cause drowsiness. Use caution when performing tasks that require alertness. May darken urine or sweat, which is not harmful. | To avoid stomach upset, take with food. | |
| **Pergolide**<br>**Mesylate**<br>*Permax* tablet (℞) | Nausea, diarrhea, constipation, confusion, low blood pressure, sweating, orthostatic hypotension. | May cause drowsiness. Use caution when performing tasks that require alertness. May darken urine or sweat, which is not harmful. | | |
| **Pramipexole**<br>**Dihydrochloride**<br>*Mirapex* tablet (℞) | Hallucinations, orthostatic hypotension, dizziness, insomnia, constipation. | | May be taken regardless of meals. Take with food if nausea experienced. | |

**ACTION** These medications reduce the frequency and severity of the symptoms of Parkinson's disease and drug-induced Parkinson-like symptoms. Symptoms include tremor, rigidity, posture disorders, and equilibrium disorders.

**INDICATION** Used alone or in combination with other medications for Parkinson's symptoms. These medications do not cure the cause of the symptom.

| Generic Name<br>*Brand Name* | Side Effects | Warnings | Dosing | Notes |
|---|---|---|---|---|
| **Procyclidine**<br>*Kemadrin* tablet (℞) | Nausea, constipation, disorientation, memory loss, weakness, agitation, rapid heart rate, vision changes. | May cause drowsiness. Use caution when performing tasks that require alertness. | To avoid stomach upset, take with food. | |
| **Selegiline HCl**<br>*Eldepryl* tablet (℞) | Nausea, urination changes, confusion, anxiety, orthostatic hypotension, blood pressure changes. | Avoid Tyramine-containing foods and drugs. | | |
| **Trihexyphenidyl**<br>*Artane* tablet, capsule, elixir (℞) | Nausea, constipation, disorientation, memory loss, weakness, agitation, rapid heart rate, vision changes. | May cause drowsiness. Use caution when performing tasks that require alertness. | To avoid stomach upset, take with food. | |

## Antipsychotic Agents— Phenothiazines

**ACTION** These medications affect chemical receptors in the brain that affect behavior, memory, and other psychological problems.

**INDICATION** Used to treat mental illness, depression, and behavioral problems.

**BANNED SUBSTANCES** NCAA and/or USOC may list some of these substances as banned for athletes to use.

| Generic Name<br>*Brand Name* | Side Effects | Warnings | Dosing | Notes |
|---|---|---|---|---|
| **Acetophenazine Maleate**<br>*Tindal* tablet (℞) | Nausea, constipation, anxiety, excitement, disturbed concentration, rapid pulse, chest pain, sensitivity to light. | May cause drowsiness. Use caution when performing tasks that require alertness. Alcohol may intensify these effects. | | |
| **Chlorpromazine**<br>*Thorazine* tablet, capsule, syrup, suppository (℞) | Nausea, constipation, anxiety, excitement, disturbed concentration, rapid pulse, chest pain, sensitivity to light. | May cause drowsiness. Use caution when performing tasks that require alertness. Alcohol may intensify these effects. | | Used to treat nonpsychotic anxiety, to control nausea and vomiting, and to relieve intractable hiccoughs. |
| **Fluphenazine**<br>*Permitil, Prolixin* tablet, elixir (℞) | Nausea, constipation, anxiety, excitement, disturbed concentration, rapid pulse, chest pain, sensitivity to light. | May cause drowsiness. Use caution when performing tasks that require alertness. Alcohol may intensify these effects. | | |
| **Mesoridazine**<br>*Serentil* tablet, liquid (℞) | Nausea, constipation, anxiety, excitement, disturbed concentration, rapid pulse, chest pain, sensitivity to light. | May cause drowsiness. Use caution when performing tasks that require alertness. Alcohol may intensify these effects. | | Used to treat schizophrenia, anxiety, and depression in alcoholics, and personality disorders in general. |

**ACTION** These medications affect chemical receptors in the brain that affect behavior, memory, and other psychological problems.

**INDICATION** Used to treat mental illness, depression, and behavioral problems.

**BANNED SUBSTANCES** NCAA and/or USOC may list some of these substances as banned for athletes to use.

| Generic Name<br>*Brand Name* | Side Effects | Warnings | Dosing | Notes |
|---|---|---|---|---|
| **Perphenazine**<br>*Trilafon* tablet,<br>liquid (℞) | Nausea, consti-pation, anxiety, excitement, dis-turbed concen-tration, rapid pulse, chest pain, sensitivity to light. | May cause drowsiness. Use caution when performing tasks that require alertness. Alco-hol may intensify these effects. | | Used to control severe nausea and vomiting, and for relief of intractable hiccoughs. |
| **Prochlorperazine**<br>*Compazine* tablet,<br>capsule, supposi-tory, syrup (℞) | Nausea, consti-pation, anxiety, excitement, dis-turbed concen-tration, rapid pulse, chest pain, sensitivity to light. | May cause drowsiness. Use caution when performing tasks that require alertness. Alco-hol may intensify these effects. | | Used to treat short-term anxiety, and to control nausea and vomiting. |
| **Promazine**<br>*Sparine* tablet (℞) | Nausea, consti-pation, anxiety, excitement, dis-turbed concen-tration, rapid pulse, chest pain, sensitivity to light. | May cause drowsiness. Use caution when performing tasks that require alertness. Alco-hol may intensify these effects. | | |
| **Thioridazine**<br>*Mellaril* tablet,<br>liquid, suspen-sion (℞) | Nausea, consti-pation, anxiety, excitement, dis-turbed concen-tration, rapid pulse, chest pain, sensitivity to light. | May cause drowsiness. Use caution when performing tasks that require alertness. Alco-hol may intensify these effects. | | Used to treat short-term depression with anxiety. |

Central Nervous System

**ACTION** These medications affect chemical receptors in the brain that affect behavior, memory, and other psychological problems.

**INDICATION** Used to treat mental illness, depression, and behavioral problems.

**BANNED SUBSTANCES** NCAA and/or USOC may list some of these substances as banned for athletes to use.

| Generic Name<br>*Brand Name* | Side Effects | Warnings | Dosing | Notes |
|---|---|---|---|---|
| **Trifluoperazine**<br>*Stelazine* tablet,<br>liquid (℞) | Nausea, constipation, anxiety, excitement, disturbed concentration, rapid pulse, chest pain, sensitivity to light. | May cause drowsiness. Use caution when performing tasks that require alertness. Alcohol may intensify these effects. | | Used for short-term treatment of anxiety. |

## Antipsychotic Agents—Miscellaneous

**ACTION** These medications affect chemical receptors in the brain that affect behavior, memory, and other psychological problems.

**INDICATION** Used to treat mental illness, depression, and behavioral problems.

**BANNED SUBSTANCES** NCAA and/or USOC may list some of these substances as banned for athletes to use.

| Generic Name<br>*Brand Name* | Side Effects | Warnings | Dosing | Notes |
|---|---|---|---|---|
| **Chlorprothixene**<br>*Taractan* tablet,<br>liquid (℞) | Nausea, constipation, anxiety, excitement, disturbed concentration, rapid pulse, chest pain, sensitivity to light. | May cause drowsiness. Use caution when performing tasks that require alertness. Alcohol may intensify these effects. | | Used to reduce the symptoms of mental illness. |

**ACTION** These medications affect chemical receptors in the brain that affect behavior, memory, and other psychological problems.

**INDICATION** Used to treat mental illness, depression, and behavioral problems.

**BANNED SUBSTANCES** NCAA and/or USOC may list some of these substances as banned for athletes to use.

| Generic Name<br>*Brand Name* | Side Effects | Warnings | Dosing | Notes |
|---|---|---|---|---|
| **Clozapine**<br>*Clozaril* tablet (℞) | Nausea, constipation, anxiety, seizures, tremor, vertigo, orthostatic hypotension, visual disturbances. | May cause drowsiness. Use caution when performing tasks that require alertness. | | Used for severely ill schizophrenic patients who fail on other medications. White blood cell testing is required to monitor for agranulocytosis. |
| **Haloperidol**<br>*Haldol* tablet,<br>liquid (℞) | Nausea, constipation, anxiety, excitement, disturbed concentration, rapid pulse, chest pain, sensitivity to light. | May cause drowsiness. Use caution when performing tasks that require alertness. Alcohol may intensify these effects. | | Used to reduce the symptoms of mental illness and to control symptoms of Tourette syndrome. |
| **Lithium Carbonate**<br>*Eskalith, Lithane*<br>tablet, capsule<br>(℞) | Nausea, vomiting, diarrhea, confusion, decreased blood pressure, visual disturbances, weight loss, cold fingers. | May cause drowsiness. Use caution when performing tasks that require alertness. Alcohol may intensify these effects. Side effects may be early signs of toxicity. | Take immediately after meals to avoid stomach upset. | Used to treat manic-depressive illness, cluster headaches, eating disorders. |

Central Nervous System

**ACTION** These medications affect chemical receptors in the brain that affect behavior, memory, and other psychological problems.

**INDICATION** Used to treat mental illness, depression, and behavioral problems.

**BANNED SUBSTANCES** NCAA and/or USOC may list some of these substances as banned for athletes to use.

| Generic Name<br>*Brand Name* | Side Effects | Warnings | Dosing | Notes |
|---|---|---|---|---|
| **Loxapine**<br>*Loxitane* capsule, liquid (℞) | Nausea, constipation, anxiety, excitement, disturbed concentration, rapid pulse, chest pain, sensitivity to light. | May cause drowsiness, caution should be used when performing tasks that require alertness. Use with alcohol may intensify these effects. | | Used to reduce the symptoms of mental illness. |
| **Molindone**<br>*Moban* tablet, liquid (℞) | Nausea, constipation, anxiety, excitement, disturbed concentration, rapid pulse, chest pain, sensitivity to light. | May cause drowsiness. Use caution when performing tasks that require alertness. Alcohol may intensify these effects. | | Used to reduce the symptoms of mental illness. |
| **Olanzapine**<br>*Zyprexa* tablet (℞) | Headache, agitation, somnolence, insomnia, nervousness, dizziness, flu syndrome, chills, fever, rhinitis, hangover effect, malaise, increased salivation, nausea, thirst, arthritis pain, leg cramps, asthma, dry skin. | Avoid alcohol, overheating, and dehydration. | May take without regard to food. | Consult a physician or pharmacist before taking over-the-counter medications. |

**ACTION** These medications affect chemical receptors in the brain that affect behavior, memory, and other psychological problems.

**INDICATION** Used to treat mental illness, depression, and behavioral problems.

**BANNED SUBSTANCES** NCAA and/or USOC may list some of these substances as banned for athletes to use.

| Generic Name<br>*Brand Name* | Side Effects | Warnings | Dosing | Notes |
|---|---|---|---|---|
| **Pimozide**<br>*Orap* tablet (℞) | Parkinson-like symptoms, tremors, tardive dyskinesia, appetite changes, seizures, blood pressure changes, blurred vision. | May cause drowsiness. Use caution when performing tasks that require alertness. | | Used to treat Tourette syndrome. |
| **Risperidone**<br>*Risperdal* tablet (℞) | Insomnia, agitation, anxiety, somnolence, headache, extrapyramidal symptoms, constipation, nausea, dyspepsia, rhinitis, rash. | Avoid alcohol, which can further impair judgment and motor skills. May make user photosensitive to sunlight. | | Consult a physician or pharmacist before taking over-the-counter medications. |
| **Thiothixene**<br>*Navane* capsule, liquid (℞) | Nausea, constipation, anxiety, excitement, disturbed concentration, rapid pulse, chest pain, sensitivity to light. | May cause drowsiness. Use caution when performing tasks that require alertness. Alcohol may intensify these effects. | | Used to reduce the symptoms of mental illness. |

## Muscle Relaxants

**ACTION** These medications generally affect nerves that cause muscle tension or spasms. They may also work directly on the muscle or through the central nervous system.

**INDICATION** Used to relieve muscle discomfort due to strain, sprain, or other injuries. These medications are not a substitute for rest or the physical therapy needed to heal the injury.

**BANNED SUBSTANCES** NCAA and/or USOC may list some of these substances as banned for athletes to use. Caffeine is limited based on urine concentration.

| Generic Name<br>*Brand Name* | Side Effects | Warnings | Dosing | Notes |
|---|---|---|---|---|
| **Baclofen**<br>*Lioresal* tablet (℞) | Frequent urination, nausea, constipation, dizziness, weakness, low blood pressure, excessive sweating. | May cause drowsiness, caution should be used when performing tasks that require alertness. | | Used for muscle spasms resulting from disorders such as multiple sclerosis. |
| **Carisoprodol**<br>*Soma* tablet (℞) | Constipation, nausea, tremor, dizziness, sleeplessness, confusion, increased heart rate, orthostatic hypotension. | May cause drowsiness, caution should be used when performing tasks that require alertness. | Take with food to avoid stomach upset. | |
| **Carisoprodol, Aspirin**<br>*Soma Compound* tablet (℞) | Constipation, nausea, tremor, dizziness, sleeplessness, confusion, increased heart rate, orthostatic hypotension. | May cause drowsiness. Use caution when performing tasks that require alertness. | Take with food to avoid stomach upset. | |
| **Carisoprodol, Aspirin, Codeine**<br>*Soma Compound with Codeine* tablet (℞, C-III) | Constipation, nausea, tremor, dizziness, sleeplessness, confusion, increased heart rate, orthostatic hypotension. | May cause drowsiness. Use caution when performing tasks that require alertness. Alcohol and other depressants may intensify this effect. | Take with food to avoid stomach upset. | |

**ACTION** These medications generally affect nerves that cause muscle tension or spasms. They may also work directly on the muscle or through the central nervous system.

**INDICATION** Used to relieve muscle discomfort due to strain, sprain, or other injuries. These medications are not a substitute for rest or the physical therapy needed to heal the injury.

**BANNED SUBSTANCES** NCAA and/or USOC may list some of these substances as banned for athletes to use. Caffeine is limited based on urine concentration.

| Generic Name<br>*Brand Name* | Side Effects | Warnings | Dosing | Notes |
|---|---|---|---|---|
| **Chlorzoxazone**<br>*Paraflex,*<br>*Parafon Forte DSC*<br>tablet (℞) | Constipation, nausea, tremor, dizziness, sleeplessness, confusion, increased heart rate, orthostatic hypotension. | May cause drowsiness. Use caution when performing tasks that require alertness. May discolor urine. | Take with food to avoid stomach upset. | |
| **Cyclobenzaprine**<br>*Flexeril* tablet (℞) | Constipation, nausea, tremor, dizziness, sleeplessness, confusion, increased heart rate, orthostatic hypotension. | May cause drowsiness. Use caution when performing tasks that require alertness. | Take with food to avoid stomach upset. | |
| **Dantrolene Sodium**<br>*Dantrium* capsule (℞) | Frequent urination, diarrhea, constipation, dizziness, seizures, blood pressure changes, swelling, vision problems. | May cause drowsiness. Use caution when performing tasks that require alertness. May make user more sensitive to sunlight. | | Used for muscle spasms resulting from disorders such as multiple sclerosis, cerebral palsy, and stroke. |
| **Metaxalone**<br>*Skelaxin* tablet (℞) | Constipation, nausea, tremor, dizziness, sleeplessness, confusion, increased heart rate, orthostatic hypotension. | May cause drowsiness. Use caution when performing tasks that require alertness. | Take with food to avoid stomach upset. | |

**ACTION** These medications generally affect nerves that cause muscle tension or spasms. They may also work directly on the muscle or through the central nervous system.

**INDICATION** Used to relieve muscle discomfort due to strain, sprain, or other injuries. These medications are not a substitute for rest or the physical therapy needed to heal the injury.

**BANNED SUBSTANCES** NCAA and/or USOC may list some of these substances as banned for athletes to use. Caffeine is limited based on urine concentration.

| Generic Name<br>*Brand Name* | Side Effects | Warnings | Dosing | Notes |
|---|---|---|---|---|
| **Methocarbamol**<br>*Robaxin* tablet (℞) | Constipation, nausea, tremor, dizziness, sleeplessness, confusion, increased heart rate, orthostatic hypotension. | May cause drowsiness. Use caution when performing tasks that require alertness. May discolor urine. | Take with food to avoid stomach upset. | |
| **Methocarbamol, Aspirin**<br>*Robaxisal* tablet (℞) | Constipation, nausea, tremor, dizziness, sleeplessness, confusion, increased heart rate, orthostatic hypotension. | May cause drowsiness. Use caution when performing tasks that require alertness. May discolor urine. | Take with food to avoid stomach upset. | |
| **Orphenadrine Citrate**<br>*Norflex* tablet (℞) | Constipation, nausea, tremor, dizziness, sleeplessness, confusion, increased heart rate, orthostatic hypotension. | May cause drowsiness. Use caution when performing tasks that require alertness. | Take with food to avoid stomach upset. | |
| **Orphenadrine Citrate, Aspirin, Caffeine**<br>*Norgesic, Norgesic Forte* tablet (℞) | Constipation, nausea, tremor, dizziness, sleeplessness, confusion, increased heart rate, orthostatic hypotension. | May cause drowsiness. Use caution when performing tasks that require alertness. | Take with food to avoid stomach upset. | Caffeine may cause nervousness and excitement. |

**ACTION** These medications generally affect nerves that cause muscle tension or spasms. They may also work directly on the muscle or through the central nervous system.

**INDICATION** Used to relieve muscle discomfort due to strain, sprain, or other injuries. These medications are not a substitute for rest or the physical therapy needed to heal the injury.

**BANNED SUBSTANCES** NCAA and/or USOC may list some of these substances as banned for athletes to use. Caffeine is limited based on urine concentration.

| Generic Name<br>*Brand Name* | Side Effects | Warnings | Dosing | Notes |
|---|---|---|---|---|
| **Tizanidine**<br>*Zanaflex* tablet (℞) | Hypotension, drowsiness, fatigue, dizziness, anxiety, nausea, vomiting. | May cause drowsiness. Use caution when performing tasks that require alertness. Alcohol and other depressants may intensify this effect. | | Used for muscle spasticity states. |

## Sedatives—Barbiturates

**ACTION** Barbiturates produce CNS mood alterations ranging from excitation to sedation. Some are useful for their anticonvulsant activity. Alcohol and other depressants will intensify side effects.

**INDICATION** Used for the short-term treatment of insomnia. Barbiturates lose their sleep-inducing effectiveness after 2 weeks.

| Generic Name<br>*Brand Name* | Side Effects | Warnings | Dosing | Notes |
|---|---|---|---|---|
| **Amobarbital**<br>*Amytal* tablet, capsule (℞, C-II) | Nausea, vomiting, agitation, confusion, nervousness, decreased blood pressure, difficult breathing, pain. | May decrease alertness. Use caution when performing tasks that require physical dexterity. | Do not use longer than 2 weeks as a sleep aid. | |

Central Nervous System

**ACTION** Barbiturates produce CNS mood alterations ranging from excitation to sedation. Some are useful for their anticonvulsant activity. Alcohol and other depressants will intensify side effects.

**INDICATION** Used for the short-term treatment of insomnia. Barbiturates lose their sleep-inducing effectiveness after 2 weeks.

| Generic Name<br>*Brand Name* | Side Effects | Warnings | Dosing | Notes |
|---|---|---|---|---|
| **Butabarbital Sodium**<br>*Butisol, Buticaps*<br>tablet, capsule, elixir (℞, C-III) | Nausea, vomiting, agitation, confusion, nervousness, decreased blood pressure, difficult breathing, pain. | May decrease alertness. Use caution when performing tasks that require physical dexterity. | Do not use longer than 2 weeks as a sleep aid. | |
| **Mephobarbital**<br>*Mebaral* tablet (℞, C-IV) | Nausea, vomiting, agitation, confusion, nervousness, decreased blood pressure, difficult breathing, pain. | May decrease alertness. Use caution when performing tasks that require physical dexterity. | Do not use longer than 2 weeks as a sleep aid. | Also used as a long-term anticonvulsant. |
| **Pentobarbital**<br>*Nembutal* capsule, elixir, suppository (℞, C-II) | Nausea, vomiting, agitation, confusion, nervousness, decreased blood pressure, difficult breathing, pain. | May decrease alertness. Use caution when performing tasks that require physical dexterity. | Do not use longer than 2 weeks as a sleep aid. | |
| **Phenobarbital**<br>*Phenobarbital* tablet, capsule, elixir (℞, C-IV) | Nausea, vomiting, agitation, confusion, nervousness, difficult breathing, pain. | May decrease alertness. Use caution when performing tasks that require physical dexterity. | Do not use longer than 2 weeks as a sleep aid. | Also used as a long-term anticonvulsant. |
| **Secobarbital**<br>*Seconal* tablet, capsule (℞, C-II) | Nausea, vomiting, agitation, confusion, nervousness, decreased blood pressure, difficult breathing, pain. | May decrease alertness. Use caution when performing tasks that require physical dexterity. | Do not use longer than 2 weeks as a sleep aid. | |

# Sedatives—Benzodiazepines

**ACTION** These benzodiazepine sedatives decrease sleep latency and the number of awakenings. If discontinued after 3 to 4 weeks patient may experience REM rebound.

**INDICATION** Used to treat insomnia characterized by difficulty in falling asleep, frequent awakenings, or early morning awakenings. Prolonged administration is not recommended.

| Generic Name<br>*Brand Name* | Side Effects | Warnings | Dosing | Notes |
|---|---|---|---|---|
| **Estazolam**<br>*Prosom* tablet<br>(℞, C-IV) | Nausea, vomiting, agitation, confusion, nervousness, decreased blood pressure, difficult breathing, pain. | May decrease alertness. Use caution when performing tasks that require physical dexterity. Avoid alcohol and other depressants. | Do not use longer than 2 weeks as a sleep aid. | Used to treat insomnia for a short period of time (1 to 2 weeks). |
| **Flurazepam**<br>*Dalmane* capsule<br>(℞, C-IV) | Nausea, vomiting, agitation, confusion, nervousness, decreased blood pressure, difficult breathing, pain. | May decrease alertness. Use caution when performing tasks that require physical dexterity. Avoid alcohol and other depressants. | Do not use longer than 2 weeks as a sleep aid. | Used to treat insomnia for a short period of time (1 to 2 weeks). |
| **Quazepam**<br>*Doral* tablet<br>(℞, C-IV) | Nausea, vomiting, agitation, confusion, nervousness, decreased blood pressure, difficult breathing, pain. | May decrease alertness. Use caution when performing tasks that require physical dexterity. Avoid alcohol and other depressants. | Do not use longer than 2 weeks as a sleep aid. | Used to treat insomnia for a short period of time (1 to 2 weeks). |
| **Temazepam**<br>*Restoril* capsule<br>(℞, C-IV) | Nausea, vomiting, agitation, confusion, nervousness, decreased blood pressure, difficult breathing, pain. | May decrease alertness. Use caution when performing tasks that require physical dexterity. Avoid alcohol and other depressants. | Do not use longer than 2 weeks as a sleep aid. | Used to treat insomnia for a short period of time (1 to 2 weeks). |

Central Nervous System

**ACTION** These benzodiazepine sedatives decrease sleep latency and the number of awakenings. If discontinued after 3 to 4 weeks patient may experience REM rebound.

**INDICATION** Used to treat insomnia characterized by difficulty in falling asleep, frequent awakenings, or early morning awakenings. Prolonged administration is not recommended.

| Generic Name<br>*Brand Name* | Side Effects | Warnings | Dosing | Notes |
|---|---|---|---|---|
| **Triazolam**<br>*Halcion* tablet<br>(℞, C-IV) | Nausea, vomiting, agitation, confusion, nervousness, decreased blood pressure, difficult breathing, pain. | May decrease alertness. Use caution when performing tasks that require physical dexterity. Avoid alcohol and other depressants. | Do not use longer than 2 weeks as a sleep aid. | Used to treat insomnia for a short period of time (1 to 2 weeks). |

## Sedatives—Miscellaneous

**ACTION** These medications produce different levels of CNS mood changes, ranging from excitement to sedation and sleep. Some may decrease the severity and frequency of seizures.

**INDICATION** Used to treat insomnia and/or seizures.

| Generic Name<br>*Brand Name* | Side Effects | Warnings | Dosing | Notes |
|---|---|---|---|---|
| **Chloral Hydrate**<br>*Noctec* capsule,<br>syrup (℞, C-IV) | Nausea, vomiting, agitation, confusion, nervousness, decreased blood pressure, difficult breathing, pain. | May decrease alertness. Use caution when performing tasks that require physical dexterity. Avoid alcohol and other depressants. | Take with a full glass of water or juice. Do not use longer than 2 weeks as a sleep aid. | Used to treat insomnia for a short period of time (1 to 2 weeks). |

**ACTION** These medications produce different levels of CNS mood changes, ranging from excitement to sedation and sleep. Some may decrease the severity and frequency of seizures.

**INDICATION** Used to treat insomnia and/or seizures.

| Generic Name<br>Brand Name | Side Effects | Warnings | Dosing | Notes |
|---|---|---|---|---|
| **Diphenhydramine**<br>*Sominex, Nytol,*<br>*Compoz* tablet<br>(OTC) | Blurred vision, dry mouth, confusion, constipation. | May decrease alertness. Use caution when performing tasks that require physical dexterity. Avoid alcohol and other depressants. | | As an antihistamine, this drug is used to treat insomnia. |
| **Doxylamine**<br>*Unisom* tablet<br>(OTC) | Blurred vision, dry mouth, confusion, constipation. | May decrease alertness. Use caution when performing tasks that require physical dexterity. Avoid alcohol and other depressants. | | As an antihistamine, this drug is used to treat insomnia. |
| **Ethchlorvynol**<br>*Placidyl* capsule<br>(℞, C-IV) | Nausea, vomiting, agitation, confusion, nervousness, decreased blood pressure, difficult breathing, pain. | May decrease alertness. Use caution when performing tasks that require physical dexterity. Avoid alcohol and other depressants. | Do not use longer than 2 weeks as a sleep aid. | Used to treat insomnia for a short period of time (1 to 2 weeks). |
| **Zolpidem Tartrate**<br>*Ambien* tablet<br>(℞, C-IV) | Nausea, vomiting, agitation, confusion, nervousness, decreased blood pressure, difficult breathing, pain. | May decrease alertness. Use caution when performing tasks that require physical dexterity. Avoid alcohol and other depressants. | Do not use longer than 2 weeks as a sleep aid. | Used to treat insomnia for a short period of time (1 to 2 weeks). |

## Stimulants—Amphetamines

**ACTION** Produce appetite suppression by a direct stimulant effect on the brain. These medications can produce drug dependence.

**INDICATION** As a short-term adjunct in a regimen of weight reduction. Some may be used for narcolepsy and Attention Deficit Disorder (ADD) with hyperactivity.

| Generic Name<br>*Brand Name* | Side Effects | Warnings | Dosing | Notes |
|---|---|---|---|---|
| **Amphetamine Mixture**<br>*Adderall* tablet<br>(℞, C-II) | Nervousness, restlessness, dizziness, insomnia, anorexia, dry mouth, GI disturbances. | May impair ability to perform tasks requiring alertness. May mask extreme fatigue. | | |
| **Amphetamine Complex**<br>*Biphetamine* capsule (℞, C-II) | Nervousness, restlessness, dizziness, insomnia, anorexia, dry mouth, GI disturbances. | May impair ability to perform tasks requiring alertness. May mask extreme fatigue. | | |
| **Dextroamphetamine Sulfate**<br>*Dexedrine* tablet, sustained release capsule (℞, C-II) | Nervousness, restlessness, dizziness, insomnia, anorexia, dry mouth, GI disturbances. | May impair ability to perform tasks requiring alertness. May mask extreme fatigue. | | |
| **Methamphetamine HCL**<br>*Desoxyn* tablet (℞, C-II) | Nervousness, restlessness, dizziness, insomnia, anorexia, dry mouth, GI disturbances. | May impair ability to perform tasks requiring alertness. May mask extreme fatigue. | | |

# Stimulants—Anorexiants

**ACTION** Produce appetite suppression by a direct stimulant effect on the satiety center of the brain. These products are pharmacologically similar to amphetamines.

**INDICATION** As a short-term adjunct in a regimen of weight reduction.

| Generic Name<br>*Brand Name* | Side Effects | Warnings | Dosing | Notes |
|---|---|---|---|---|
| **Benzphetamine**<br>**HCl**<br>*Didrex* tablet<br>(R, C-III) | Insomnia, dry mouth, constipation, dizziness, fatigue, depression. | | | |
| **Dexfenfluramine**<br>*Redux* capsule<br>(R, C-IV) | Insomnia, dry mouth, constipation, dizziness, fatigue, depression. | | | **Withdrawn from market in September 1997 due to potential to instigate heart valve problems.** |
| **Diethylpropion**<br>**HCl**<br>*Tenuate* tablet, sustained-release tablet (R, C-IV) | Insomnia, dry mouth, constipation, dizziness, fatigue, depression. | | Take 1 hour before meal | |
| **Fenfluramine HCl**<br>*Pondimin* tablet<br>(R, C-IV) | Insomnia, dry mouth, constipation, dizziness, fatigue, depression, pulmonary hypertension. | Alcohol may intensify drowsiness. | | **Withdrawn from market in September 1997 due to potential to instigate heart valve problems.** |
| **Mazindol**<br>*Sanorex, Mazanor* tablet (R, C-V) | Insomnia, dry mouth, constipation, dizziness, fatigue, depression. | | May be taken with meals to reduce GI irritation. | |
| **Phendimetrazine**<br>**Tartrate**<br>*Bontril PDM* tablet<br>(R, C-III)<br>*Bontril* capsule<br>(R, C-III) | Insomnia, dry mouth, constipation, dizziness, fatigue, depression. | | Take 1 hour before meal. | |

Central Nervous System

**ACTION** Produce appetite suppression by a direct stimulant effect on the satiety center of the brain. These products are pharmacologically similar to amphetamines.

**INDICATION** As a short-term adjunct in a regimen of weight reduction.

| Generic Name<br>Brand Name | Side Effects | Warnings | Dosing | Notes |
|---|---|---|---|---|
| **Phenmetrazine HCl**<br>*Preludin* sustained-release tablet<br>(℞, C-II) | Insomnia, dry mouth, constipation, dizziness, fatigue, depression. | | | |
| **Phentermine HCl**<br>*Fastin, Adipex-P* capsule (℞, C-IV)<br>*Adipex-P* tablet<br>(℞, C-IV) | Insomnia, dry mouth, constipation, dizziness, fatigue, depression. | | Take 30 minutes before meal. | |
| **Phentermine Resin**<br>*Ionamin* capsule<br>(℞, C-IV) | Insomnia, dry mouth, constipation, dizziness, fatigue, depression. | | | |

## Stimulants—Miscellaneous

**ACTION** Produce appetite suppression by a variety of stimulant effects.

**INDICATION** As a short-term adjunct in a regimen of weight reduction.

**BANNED SUBSTANCES** NCAA and/or USOC may list some of these substances as banned for athletes to use.

| Generic Name<br>Brand Name | Side Effects | Warnings | Dosing | Notes |
|---|---|---|---|---|
| **Caffeine**<br>*NoDoz, Vivarin* tablet (OTC) | Insomnia, restlessness, excitement, nausea, stomach pain, diuresis. | Headache, anxiety, and muscle tension may be result of withdrawal symptoms. | | Drug may be found in combination with other medications. |

**ACTION** Produce appetite suppression by a variety of stimulant effects.

**INDICATION** As a short-term adjunct in a regimen of weight reduction.

**BANNED SUBSTANCES** NCAA and/or USOC may list some of these substances as banned for athletes to use.

| Generic Name<br>Brand Name | Side Effects | Warnings | Dosing | Notes |
|---|---|---|---|---|
| **Phenylpropa-<br>nolamine HCL**<br>Dexatrim capsule<br>(OTC),<br>Acutrim tablet<br>(OTC) | Palpitations,<br>tachycardia,<br>restlessness,<br>dizziness, insom-<br>nia, headache,<br>nasal dryness,<br>dry mouth. | | Do not exceed<br>recommended<br>dose. | Drug may be<br>found in some<br>cough and cold<br>products. |

## Miscellaneous CNS Agents

**ACTION** These medications affect chemical receptors in the brain that affect behavior, memory, and other psychological problems.

**INDICATION** Used to treat mental illness, depression, and behavioral problems.

**BANNED SUBSTANCES** NCAA and/or USOC may list some of these substances as banned for athletes to use.

| Generic Name<br>Brand Name | Side Effects | Warnings | Dosing | Notes |
|---|---|---|---|---|
| **Donepezil HCl**<br>Aricept tablet (℞) | Nausea, diarrhea,<br>vomiting. | Contact a physi-<br>cian if fainting,<br>difficult breath-<br>ing, severe<br>sweating, or sa-<br>livation occurs. | For best thera-<br>peutic progress,<br>do not skip<br>doses. | Used for<br>treatment of<br>Alzheimer's<br>disease. |
| **Ergoloid<br>Mesylate**<br>Hydergine, Gerimal<br>tablet, capsule,<br>liquid (℞) | Nausea,<br>stomach upset. | | Treatment may<br>take 6 months to<br>determine<br>effectiveness. | Used to treat<br>age-related<br>decrease in<br>mental ability<br>sometimes as-<br>sociated with<br>Alzheimer's<br>disease, demen-<br>tia, or stroke. |

Central Nervous System

**ACTION** These medications affect chemical receptors in the brain that affect behavior, memory, and other psychological problems.

**INDICATION** Used to treat mental illness, depression, and behavioral problems.

**BANNED SUBSTANCES** NCAA and/or USOC may list some of these substances as banned for athletes to use.

| Generic Name<br>*Brand Name* | Side Effects | Warnings | Dosing | Notes |
|---|---|---|---|---|
| **Methylphenidate HCl**<br>*Ritalin, Ritalin-SR* tablet (℞, C-II) | Appetite loss, nausea, nervousness, sleeplessness, headache, chest pain. | May impair co-ordination. Use caution when performing tasks that require physical dexterity. | | Used to treat Attention Deficit Disorder (ADD), hyperactivity, and narcolepsy. |
| **Pemoline**<br>*Cylert* (℞, C-IV) | Appetite loss, weight loss, nausea, seizures, irritability, depression. | May cause dizziness. Use caution when performing tasks that require alertness. | | Used to treat Attention Deficit Disorder (ADD), hyperactivity, and narcolepsy. |
| **Tacrine HCl**<br>*Cognex* capsule (℞) | Nausea, vomiting, diarrhea, rash, jaundice. | It important to maintain a regular dosing schedule. | Take between meals; however, may take with meals to reduce GI upset. | Treats mild to moderate Alzheimer-type dementia. |

# Metabolic Agents

## Corticosteroids

**ACTION** Hormones produced by the pituitary and adrenal glands affect kidney function, the immune system, and the inflammatory response by the body; calcitonin affects bone mass.

**INDICATION** For a variety of purposes including respiratory problems, inflammatory conditions, allergic conditions, dermatologic conditions, and collagen disorders.

**BANNED SUBSTANCES** NCAA and/or USOC may list some of these substances as banned for athletes to use.

| Generic Name<br>*Brand Name* | Side Effects | Warnings | Dosing | Notes |
|---|---|---|---|---|
| **Betamethasone**<br>*Celestone* tablet,<br>syrup (℞) | Nausea, vomiting, behavior changes, low blood pressure, acne; long-term effects include moon-face and weight gain. | Avoid rapid withdrawal of therapy if used long term. | May take with meals to avoid stomach upset. | |
| **Cortisone**<br>*Cortisone* tablet<br>(℞) | Nausea, vomiting, behavior changes, low blood pressure, acne; long-term effects include moon face and weight gain. | Avoid rapid withdrawal of therapy if used long term. | May take with meals to avoid stomach upset. | |
| **Dexamethasone**<br>*Decadron,*<br>*Hexadrol* tablet,<br>elixir (℞) | Nausea, vomiting, behavior changes, low blood pressure, acne; long-term effects include moon face and weight gain. | Avoid rapid withdrawal of therapy if used long term. | May take with meals to avoid stomach upset. | |

**ACTION** Hormones produced by the pituitary and adrenal glands affect kidney function, the immune system, and the inflammatory response by the body; calcitonin affects bone mass.

**INDICATION** For a variety of purposes including respiratory problems, inflammatory conditions, allergic conditions, dermatologic conditions, and collagen disorders.

**BANNED SUBSTANCES** NCAA and/or USOC may list some of these substances as banned for athletes to use.

| Generic Name<br>Brand Name | Side Effects | Warnings | Dosing | Notes |
|---|---|---|---|---|
| **Fludrocortisone Acetate**<br>Florinef tablet (℞) | High blood pressure, heart failure, edema, weight gain, muscle weakness. | Do not stop taking suddenly. | | Mineralocorticoid used to treat Addison's disease and excessive salt loss. |
| **Hydrocortisone**<br>Cortef, Hydrocortisone, Cortenema tablet, enema, suspension (℞) | Nausea, vomiting, behavior changes, low blood pressure, acne; long-term effects include moon face and weight gain. | Avoid rapid withdrawal of therapy if used long term. | May take with meals to avoid stomach upset. | |
| **Methylprednisolone**<br>Medrol tablet (℞) | Nausea, vomiting, behavior changes, low blood pressure, acne; long-term effects include moon-face and weight gain. | Avoid rapid withdrawal of therapy if used long term. | May take with meals to avoid stomach upset. | |
| **Prednisone**<br>Deltasone, Orasone, Sterapred tablet, solution (℞) | Nausea, vomiting, behavior changes, low blood pressure, acne; long-term effects include moon-face and weight gain. | Avoid rapid withdrawal of therapy if used long term. | May take with meals to avoid stomach upset. | |

**ACTION** Hormones produced by the pituitary and adrenal glands affect kidney function, the immune system, and the inflammatory response by the body; calcitonin affects bone mass.

**INDICATION** For a variety of purposes including respiratory problems, inflammatory conditions, allergic conditions, dermatologic conditions, and collagen disorders.

**BANNED SUBSTANCES** NCAA and/or USOC may list some of these substances as banned for athletes to use.

| Generic Name<br>*Brand Name* | Side Effects | Warnings | Dosing | Notes |
|---|---|---|---|---|
| **Prednisolone**<br>*Delta-Cortef,*<br>*Prelone, Pedia-Pred*<br>tablet, syrup,<br>liquid (℞) | Nausea, vomiting, behavior changes, low blood pressure, acne; long-term effects include moon-face and weight gain. | Avoid rapid withdrawal of therapy if used long term. | May take with meals to avoid stomach upset. | |
| **Triamcinolone**<br>*Aristocort,*<br>*Kenacort* tablet,<br>syrup (℞) | Nausea, vomiting, behavior changes, low blood pressure, acne; long-term effects include moon-face and weight gain. | Avoid rapid withdrawal of therapy if used long term. | May take with meals to avoid stomach upset. | |

## Diabetic Agents

**ACTION** The pancreases produces insulin, which is the primary hormone that regulates blood glucose levels. Medications affect glucose levels by either changing insulin levels or glucose levels.

**INDICATION** Hypoglycemia (low blood sugar) or hyperglycemia (high blood sugar).

| Generic Name<br>*Brand Name* | Side Effects | Warnings | Dosing | Notes |
|---|---|---|---|---|
| **Acarbose**<br>*Precose* tablet (℞) | Stomach pain, diarrhea, gas. | Be sure to follow diet, exercise, and glucose-testing regimen. | Take with the first bite of each main meal. | Used to delay and reduce absorption of glucose to decrease blood sugar levels. |

Metabolic

**ACTION** The pancreases produces insulin, which is the primary hormone that regulates blood glucose levels. Medications affect glucose levels by either changing insulin levels or glucose levels.

**INDICATION** Hypoglycemia (low blood sugar) or hyperglycemia (high blood sugar).

| Generic Name Brand Name | Side Effects | Warnings | Dosing | Notes |
|---|---|---|---|---|
| **Acetohexamide** Dymelor tablet (R) | Increased heart rate, hypoglycemia, nausea, diarrhea, fatigue, eczema, sensitivity to sunlight. | Be sure to follow diet, exercise, and glucose-testing regimen. Avoid alcohol as it can cause changes in blood sugar and flushing. | May take with food if causes stomach upset. | Sulfonylurea agents decrease blood sugar by stimulating release of insulin from the pancreas. |
| **Chlorpropamide** Diabinese tablet (R) | Increased heart rate, hypoglycemia, nausea, diarrhea, fatigue, eczema, sensitivity to sunlight, vomiting. | Be sure to follow diet, exercise, and glucose-testing regimen. Avoid alcohol as it can cause changes in blood sugar and flushing. | May take with food if causes stomach upset. | Sulfonylurea agents decrease blood sugar by stimulating release of insulin from the pancreas. |
| **Diazoxide** Proglycem capsule, suspension (R) | Fluid retention, anorexia, nausea, abdominal pain, diarrhea, headache. | Monitor urine for glucose and ketones. | | Management of hypoglycemia due to hyperinsulinism. |
| **Glimepiride** Amaryl tablet (R) | Hypoglycemia, dizziness, asthenia, headache, nausea. | Be sure to follow diet, exercise, and glucose-testing regimen. Avoid alcohol as it can cause changes in blood sugar and flushing. | Take with breakfast or the first meal of the day. | |

**ACTION** The pancreases produces insulin, which is the primary hormone that regulates blood glucose levels. Medications affect glucose levels by either changing insulin levels or glucose levels.

**INDICATION** Hypoglycemia (low blood sugar) or hyperglycemia (high blood sugar).

| Generic Name<br>*Brand Name* | Side Effects | Warnings | Dosing | Notes |
|---|---|---|---|---|
| **Glipizide**<br>*Glucotrol,*<br>*Glucotrol XL*<br>tablet (℞) | Increased heart rate, hypoglycemia, nausea, diarrhea, fatigue, eczema, sensitivity to sunlight. | Be sure to follow diet, exercise, and glucose-testing regimen. Avoid alcohol as it can cause changes in blood sugar and flushing. | May take with food if causes stomach upset. Take *Glucotrol XL* at least 30 minutes before eating. | Sulfonylurea agents decrease blood sugar by stimulating release of insulin from the pancreas. |
| **Glyburide**<br>*Diabeta,*<br>*Micronase, Glynase*<br>tablet (℞) | Increased heart rate, hypoglycemia, nausea, diarrhea, fatigue, eczema, sensitivity to sunlight. | Be sure to follow diet, exercise, and glucose-testing regimen. Avoid alcohol as it can cause changes in blood sugar and flushing. | May take with food if causes stomach upset. | Sulfonylurea agents decrease blood sugar by stimulating release of insulin from the pancreas. |
| **Insulin**<br>*Humulin, Novolin*<br>injection (OTC)<br>*Humalog* injection<br>(℞) | Visual changes, skin puckering at injection site. | Blood sugar can be affected by diet, exercise, and other illnesses. Monitoring of blood sugar is imperative to avoid long-term complications of diabetes. | | Comes in short-acting, medium-acting, and long-acting forms. |
| **Metformin HCl**<br>*Glucophage* tablet<br>(℞) | Muscle pain, stomach pain, slow heartbeat, weakness, diarrhea, nausea, appetite loss, metallic taste. | Be sure to follow diet, exercise, and glucose-testing regimen. Avoid alcohol as it can cause changes in blood sugar and flushing. | Take with meals. | Improves glucose tolerance by lowering blood sugar levels. It enhances insulin sensitivity and reduces absorption of glucose. |

Metabolic

**ACTION** The pancreases produces insulin, which is the primary hormone that regulates blood glucose levels. Medications affect glucose levels by either changing insulin levels or glucose levels.

**INDICATION** Hypoglycemia (low blood sugar) or hyperglycemia (high blood sugar).

| Generic Name<br>*Brand Name* | Side Effects | Warnings | Dosing | Notes |
|---|---|---|---|---|
| **Miglitol**<br>*Glyset* tablet (℞) | Flatulence, soft stools, diarrhea, abdominal pain. | Be sure to follow diet, exercise, and glucose testing regimen. | Take with the first bite of each main meal. | Used to delay and reduce absorption of glucose to decrease blood sugar levels. |
| **Tolazamide**<br>*Tolinase* tablet (℞) | Increased heart rate, hypoglycemia, nausea, diarrhea, fatigue, eczema, sensitivity to sunlight. | Be sure to follow diet, exercise, and glucose-testing regimen. Avoid alcohol as it can cause changes in blood sugar and flushing. | May take with food if causes stomach upset. | Sulfonylurea agents decrease blood sugar by stimulating release of insulin from the pancreas. |
| **Tolbutamide**<br>*Orinase* tablet (℞) | Increased heart rate, hypoglycemia, nausea, diarrhea, fatigue, eczema, sensitivity to sunlight. | Be sure to follow diet, exercise, and glucose-testing regimen. Avoid alcohol as it can cause changes in blood sugar and flushing. | May take with food if causes stomach upset. | Sulfonylurea agents decrease blood sugar by stimulating release of insulin from the pancreas. |
| **Troglitazone**<br>*Rezulin* tablet (℞) | Dizziness, edema, hypoglycemia, nausea, vomiting, abdominal fullness, epigastritis, diarrhea. | During periods of stress such as fever, infection, or surgery, insulin requirements may change. | Take with food to enhance absorption. If a dose is missed, take it with the next meal. | Used only in patients who receive insulin. |

# Hormones—Anabolic & Androgenic

**ACTION** Anabolic steroids promote body tissue-building processes and reverse destructive tissue-depleting processes. Anabolic steroids decrease normal testosterone release. Androgen steroids are male sex hormones that promote normal growth and development of male sex organs and affect fertility.

**INDICATION** Anabolic steroids are used to treat weight loss due to severe illness and androgenic steroids are used to treat testosterone deficiency and male impotence.

**BANNED SUBSTANCES** NCAA and/or USOC may list some of these substances as banned for athletes to use.

| Generic Name<br>*Brand Name* | Side Effects | Warnings | Dosing | Notes |
|---|---|---|---|---|
| **Fluoxymesterone**<br>*Halotestin* tablet<br>(℞, C-III) | Sex drive changes, anxiety, depression, increased cholesterol, liver problems, depression, acne; Males: breast enlargement, erection problems; Females: menstrual changes. | Some adverse effects are irreversible. Androgens should not be used to enhance physical performance. | | |
| **Methyltesto-**<br>**sterone**<br>*Android, Oreton,*<br>*Testred* tablet,<br>capsule (℞, C-III) | Sex drive changes, anxiety, depression, increased cholesterol, liver problems, depression, acne; Males: breast enlargement, erection problems; Females: menstrual changes. | Some adverse effects are irreversible. Androgens should not be used to enhance physical performance. | | |

Metabolic

**ACTION** Anabolic steroids promote body tissue-building processes and reverse destructive tissue-depleting processes. Anabolic steroids decrease normal testosterone release. Androgen steroids are male sex hormones that promote normal growth and development of male sex organs and affect fertility.

**INDICATION** Anabolic steroids are used to treat weight loss due to severe illness and androgenic steroids are used to treat testosterone deficiency and male impotence.

**BANNED SUBSTANCES** NCAA and/or USOC may list some of these substances as banned for athletes to use.

| Generic Name<br>*Brand Name* | Side Effects | Warnings | Dosing | Notes |
|---|---|---|---|---|
| **Oxandrolone**<br>*Oxandrin* tablet<br>(℞, C-III) | Sex drive changes, behavioral disturbances, liver disease, depression, dependency; Males: breast enlargement, impotence, prostrate problems; Females: body hair growth, menstrual changes. | Some adverse effects are irreversible. Do not use to enhance physical performance. | | Effect of anabolic steroids may persist for 6 months after last dose. |
| **Oxymetholone**<br>*Anadrol* tablet<br>(℞, C-III) | Sex drive changes, behavioral disturbances, liver disease, depression, dependency; Males: breast enlargement, impotence, prostrate problems; Females: body hair growth, menstrual changes. | Some adverse effects are irreversible. Do not use to enhance physical performance. | | Effect of anabolic steroids may persist for 6 months after last dose. |

**ACTION** Anabolic steroids promote body tissue-building processes and reverse destructive tissue-depleting processes. Anabolic steroids decrease normal testosterone release. Androgen steroids are male sex hormones that promote normal growth and development of male sex organs and affect fertility.

**INDICATION** Anabolic steroids are used to treat weight loss due to severe illness and androgenic steroids are used to treat testosterone deficiency and male impotence.

**BANNED SUBSTANCES** NCAA and/or USOC may list some of these substances as banned for athletes to use.

| Generic Name<br>*Brand Name* | Side Effects | Warnings | Dosing | Notes |
|---|---|---|---|---|
| **Stanozolol**<br>*Winstrol* tablet<br>(℞, C-III) | Sex drive changes, behavioral disturbances, liver disease, depression, dependency; Males: breast enlargement, impotence, prostrate problems; Females: body hair growth, menstrual changes. | Some adverse effects are irreversible. Do not use to enhance physical performance. | | Effect of anabolic steroids may persist for 6 months after last dose. |
| **Testosterone**<br>*Androderm,*<br>*Testoderm*<br>transdermal patch (℞, C-III) | Sex drive changes, anxiety, depression, increased cholesterol, liver problems, depression, acne; Males: breast enlargement, erection problems; Females: menstrual changes. | Some adverse effects are irreversible. Androgens should not be used to enhance physical performance. | | |

## Hormones—Estrogens

**ACTION** Estrogens are produced by various glands, although the ovaries produce the most. They play a key role in the development and normal function of the female reproductive system.

**INDICATION** Estrogen replacement therapy is used for menopause and surgery, and for hot flashes associated with menopause.

| Generic Name<br>*Brand Name* | Side Effects | Warnings | Dosing | Notes |
|---|---|---|---|---|
| **Chlorotrianisene**<br>*Tace* capsule (℞) | Nausea, stomach cramps, painful menstruation, depression, weakness, weight changes, fluid retention, high blood pressure. | Notify a doctor if chest pain, shortness of breath, pregnancy, abdominal pain, breast lumps, or fainting occurs. | | Used to treat breast engorgement after childbirth. |
| **Conjugated Estrogens**<br>*Premarin* tablet, vaginal cream (℞) | Nausea, stomach cramps, painful menstruation, depression, weakness, weight changes, fluid retention, high blood pressure. | Notify a doctor if chest pain, shortness of breath, pregnancy, abdominal pain, breast lumps, or fainting occurs. | | Used for prevention of osteoporosis and to treat breast engorgement after childbirth. |
| **Dienestrol**<br>*DV, Ortho Dienestrol* vaginal cream (℞) | Nausea, stomach cramps, painful menstruation, depression, weakness, weight changes, fluid retention, high blood pressure. | Notify a doctor if chest pain, shortness of breath, pregnancy, abdominal pain, breast lumps, or fainting occurs. | | |
| **Diethylstilbestrol**<br>*DES* tablet (℞) | Nausea, stomach cramps, painful menstruation, depression, weakness, weight changes, fluid retention, high blood pressure. | Notify a doctor if chest pain, shortness of breath, pregnancy, abdominal pain, breast lumps, or fainting occurs. | | |

**ACTION** Estrogens are produced by various glands, although the ovaries produce the most. They play a key role in the development and normal function of the female reproductive system.

**INDICATION** Estrogen replacement therapy is used for menopause and surgery, and for hot flashes associated with menopause.

| Generic Name<br>*Brand Name* | Side Effects | Warnings | Dosing | Notes |
|---|---|---|---|---|
| **Esterified**<br>    **Estrogens**<br>*Estratab, Menest*<br>    tablet (℞) | Nausea, stomach cramps, painful menstruation, depression, weakness, weight changes, fluid retention, high blood pressure. | Notify a doctor if chest pain, shortness of breath, pregnancy, abdominal pain, breast lumps, or fainting occurs. | | |
| **Estradiol**<br>*Estrace* tablet,<br>    vaginal cream (℞)<br>*Vivelle, Climara,*<br>*Estraderm* transdermal patch (℞) | Nausea, stomach cramps, painful menstruation, depression, weakness, weight changes, fluid retention, high blood pressure. | Notify a doctor if chest pain, shortness of breath, pregnancy, abdominal pain, breast lumps, or fainting occurs. | | Used to prevent osteoporosis. |
| **Estropipate**<br>*Ogen, Ortho-Est*<br>    tablet (℞)<br>*Ogen* vaginal<br>    cream (℞) | Nausea, stomach cramps, painful menstruation, depression, weakness, weight changes, fluid retention, high blood pressure. | Notify a doctor if chest pain, shortness of breath, pregnancy, abdominal pain, breast lumps, or fainting occurs. | | |
| **Ethinyl Estradiol**<br>*Estinyl* tablet (℞) | Nausea, stomach cramps, painful menstruation, depression, weakness, weight changes, fluid retention, high blood pressure. | Notify a doctor if chest pain, shortness of breath, pregnancy, abdominal pain, breast lumps, or fainting occurs. | | |

Metabolic

**ACTION** Estrogens are produced by various glands, although the ovaries produce the most. They play a key role in the development and normal function of the female reproductive system.

**INDICATION** Estrogen replacement therapy is used for menopause and surgery, and for hot flashes associated with menopause.

| Generic Name<br>*Brand Name* | Side Effects | Warnings | Dosing | Notes |
|---|---|---|---|---|
| **Quinestrol**<br>*Estrovis* tablet (℞) | Nausea, stomach cramps, painful menstruation, depression, weakness, weight changes, fluid retention, high blood pressure. | Notify a doctor if chest pain, short-ness of breath, pregnancy, ab-dominal pain, breast lumps, or fainting occurs. | | |

## Hormones—Progestins

**ACTION** Progestins prepare the uterus for implantation of the egg and prevent ovulation.

**INDICATION** Progestins are used to treat amenorrhea, endometriosis, and abnormal uterine bleeding.

| Generic Name<br>*Brand Name* | Side Effects | Warnings | Dosing | Notes |
|---|---|---|---|---|
| **Medroxypro-gesterone**<br>*Provera, Amen, Cycrin, Curretab* tablet (℞) | Nausea, depres-sion, dizziness, numbness, men-strual flow changes, breast tenderness, fluid retention. | Notify a doctor if chest pain, short-ness of breath, pregnancy, se-vere headache, or fainting occurs. | Take with food to avoid stomach upset. | |
| **Norethindrone**<br>*Norlutin, Micronor, Nor-QD* tablet (℞) | Nausea, depres-sion, dizziness, numbness, men-strual flow changes, breast tenderness, fluid retention. | Notify a doctor if chest pain, short-ness of breath, pregnancy, se-vere headache, or fainting occurs. | Take with food to avoid stomach upset. | |

**ACTION** Progestins prepare the uterus for implantation of the egg and prevent ovulation.

**INDICATION** Progestins are used to treat amenorrhea, endometriosis, and abnormal uterine bleeding.

| Generic Name<br>Brand Name | Side Effects | Warnings | Dosing | Notes |
|---|---|---|---|---|
| **Norethindrone**<br>**Acetate**<br>*Aygestin, Norlutate*<br>tablet (℞) | Nausea, depression, dizziness, numbness, menstrual flow changes, breast tenderness, fluid retention. | Notify a doctor if chest pain, shortness of breath, pregnancy, severe headache, or fainting occurs. | Take with food to avoid stomach upset. | |

# Hormones—Combinations

Androgen, estrogen, and progestin are found in numerous combinations used to treat a variety of diseases. Some combinations are used as an oral contraceptive to prevent pregnancy and to regulate menstrual cycles. Antibiotics and other medications may decrease the effectiveness of those used as oral contraceptives.

The FDA has declared some oral contraceptive combinations safe and effective for emergency contraception taken at higher doses within 72 hours of unprotected intercourse. Ortho Tri-Cyclen has been approved for treating acne in women older than 14 when topical acne treatments have failed.

**BANNED SUBSTANCES** NCAA and/or USOC may list some of these substances as banned for athletes to use.

| Brand Name | Androgen | Estrogen | Progestin |
|---|---|---|---|
| *Alesse* | none | **Ethinyl Estradiol** | **Levonorgestrel** |
| *Demulen* | none | **Ethinyl Estradiol** | **Ethynodiol Diacetate** |
| *Desogen* | none | **Ethinyl Estradiol** | **Desogestrel** |
| *Envoid* | none | **Mestranol** | **Norethynodrel** |
| *Estratest* | **Methyltestosterone** | **Esterfied Estrogens** | none |
| *Estratest HS* | **Methyltestosterone** | **Esterfied Estrogens** | none |
| *Halodrin* | **Fluoxymesterone** | **Ethinyl Estradiol** | none |
| *Levlen* | none | **Ethinyl Estradiol** | **Levonorgestrel** |
| *Lo/Ovral* | none | **Ethinyl Estradiol** | **Norgestrol** |

Metabolic

Androgen, estrogen, and progestin are found in numerous combinations used to treat a variety of diseases. Some combinations are used as an oral contraceptive to prevent pregnancy and to regulate menstrual cycles. Antibiotics and other medications may decrease the effectiveness of those used as oral contraceptives.

The FDA has declared some oral contraceptive combinations safe and effective for emergency contraception taken at higher doses within 72 hours of unprotected intercourse. Ortho Tri-Cyclen has been approved for treating acne in women older than 14 when topical acne treatments have failed.

**BANNED SUBSTANCES** NCAA and/or USOC may list some of these substances as banned for athletes to use.

| Brand Name | Androgen | Estrogen | Progestin |
|---|---|---|---|
| Loestrin | none | Ethinyl Estradiol | Norethindrone Acetate |
| Modicon | none | Ethinyl Estradiol | Norethindrone |
| Nordette | none | Ethinyl Estradiol | Levonorgestrel |
| Norinyl 1+35 | none | Ethinyl Estradiol | Norethindrone |
| Norinyl 1+50 | none | Mestranol | Norethindrone |
| Norlestrin | none | Ethinyl Estradiol | Norethindrone Acetate |
| Ortho-Cyclen | none | Ethinyl Estradiol | Norgestimate |
| Ortho-Novum 1/35 | none | Ethinyl Estradiol | Norethindrone |
| Ortho-Novum 1/50 | none | Mestranol | Norethindrone |
| Ortho-Novum 10/11 | none | Ethinyl Estradiol | Norethindrone |
| Ortho-Novum 7/7/7 | none | Ethinyl Estradiol | Norethindrone |
| Ortho Tri-Cyclen | none | Ethinyl Estradiol | Norgestimate |
| Ovcon | none | Ethinyl Estradiol | Norethindrone |
| Ovral | none | Ethinyl Estradiol | Norgestrol |
| Ovrette | none | none | Norgestrel |
| Premarin with Methyl-testosterone | Methyltestosterone | Conjugated Estrogens | none |
| Premphase | none | Conjugated Estrogens | Medroxyproges-terone Acetate |
| Prempro | none | Conjugated Estrogens | Medroxyproges-terone Acetate |
| Tri-Levlen | none | Ethinyl Estradiol | Levonorgestrel |
| Tri-Norinyl | none | Ethinyl Estradiol | Norethindrone |
| Triphasil | none | Ethinyl Estradiol | Levonorgestrel |

## Thyroid Agents

**ACTION** Thyroid hormones increase the metabolic rate of body tissues.

**INDICATION** Medications are used either as replacement or supplemental therapy for thyroid deficiencies or to suppress thyroid production.

**BANNED SUBSTANCES** NCAA and/or USOC may list some of these substances as banned for athletes to use.

| Generic Name Brand Name | Side Effects | Warnings | Dosing | Notes |
|---|---|---|---|---|
| **Levothyroxine** Synthroid, Levoxyl, Levothroid tablet (℞) | Diarrhea, vomiting, tremors, increased heart rate, chest pain. | Replacement therapy is usually for life. | Take on an empty stomach. | Used to threat hypothyroidism (underactive thyroid). |
| **Liothyronine** Cytomel tablet (℞) | Diarrhea, vomiting, tremors, increased heart rate, chest pain. | Replacement therapy is usually for life. | Take on an empty stomach. | Used to threat hypothyroidism (underactive thyroid). |
| **Liotrix** Thyrolar tablet (℞) | Diarrhea, vomiting, tremors, increased heart rate, chest pain. | Replacement therapy is usually for life. | Take on an empty stomach. | Used to threat hypothyroidism (underactive thyroid). |
| **Methimazole** Tapazole tablet (℞) | Nausea, vomiting, depression, joint pain, edema. | | Take at regular intervals as prescribed. | Used to threat hyperthyroidism (overactive thyroid). |
| **Propylthiouracil** PTU tablet (℞) | Nausea, vomiting, depression, joint pain, edema. | | Take at regular intervals as prescribed. | Used to threat hyperthyroidism (overactive thyroid). |
| **Thyroid** Armour Thyroid tablet (℞) | Diarrhea, vomiting, tremors, increased heart rate, chest pain. | Replacement therapy is usually for life. | Take on an empty stomach. | Used to threat hypothyroidism (underactive thyroid). |

Metabolic

## Miscellaneous Metabolic Agents

**ACTION** These medications affect various metabolic systems.

**INDICATION** Used for a variety of purposes including osteoporosis, endometriosis, bed wetting, and bone disorders.

**BANNED SUBSTANCES** NCAA and/or USOC may list some of these substances as banned for athletes to use.

| Generic Name<br>*Brand Name* | Side Effects | Warnings | Dosing | Notes |
|---|---|---|---|---|
| **Alendronate Sodium**<br>*Fosamax* tablet (℞) | Nausea, ulcers, high blood pressure, rapid heartbeat, edema, fatigue, vision changes. | Supplemental calcium and vitamin D may be required. | Take 30 minutes before first food in morning with full glass of water. Do not lie down for at least 30 minutes. | Used to treat osteoporosis in women. |
| **Aminoglute-thimide**<br>*Cytadren* tablet (℞) | Drowsiness, dizziness, headache, rash, nausea, loss of appetite. | Use caution when performing tasks requiring alertness. | | Used for suppression of adrenal function in Cushing's syndrome. |
| **Calcitonin**<br>*Miacalcin, Calcimar* nasal spray, injection (℞) | Headache, anxiety, vertigo, fast heartbeat, nasal problems, visual problems. | Supplemental calcium and vitamin D may be required. | | Used to treat postmenopausal osteoporosis and problems associated with abnormal bone formation and calcium uptake. |
| **Danazol**<br>*Danocrine* capsule (℞) | Masculinity effects, flushing, sweating, vaginitis, emotional instability. | | | Used to treat endometriosis and fibrocystic breast disease. |
| **Desmopressin Acetate**<br>*DDAVP* tablet, nasal spray (℞) | Headache, nausea, stomach cramps, dizziness, chest pain. | | | Human antidiuretic hormone (ADH) used to treat excessive urination, nighttime bed-wetting, and bleeding in hemophilia. |

**ACTION** These medications affect various metabolic systems.

**INDICATION** Used for a variety of purposes including osteoporosis, endometriosis, bed wetting, and bone disorders.

**BANNED SUBSTANCES** NCAA and/or USOC may list some of these substances as banned for athletes to use.

| Generic Name<br>*Brand Name* | Side Effects | Warnings | Dosing | Notes |
|---|---|---|---|---|
| **Etidronate Disodium**<br>*Didronel* tablet (℞) | Nausea, ulcers, high blood pressure, rapid heartbeat, edema, fatigue, vision changes. | | Take 2 hours before meals with full glass of water. | Used to treat high calcium blood levels. |
| **Nafarelin Acetate**<br>*Synarel* nasal solution (℞) | Depression, headache, sleeplessness, chest pain, body odor, weight changes, edema. | Usual course of therapy is 6 months. | Wait 30 seconds between sprays. | Used for treatment of endometriosis and central precocious puberty. |
| **Tiludronate Disodium**<br>*Skelid* tablet (℞) | Nausea, diarrhea, dyspepsia. | Maintain adequate vitamin D and calcium intake. | Do not take within 2 hours of food, calcium supplements, or antacids. Take with 8 ounces of plain water. | Used for treatment of Paget's disease of the bone. |

Metabolic

# Miscellaneous

## Mouth and Throat Products

**ACTION** Reduce inflammation in the mouth and throat.

**INDICATION** Generally for cold sores, fever blisters, irritation, and inflammation.

| Generic Name<br>Brand Name | Side Effects | Warnings | Dosing | Notes |
|---|---|---|---|---|
| **Amlexanox**<br>Aphthasol oral<br>paste (℞) | Stinging, burn-<br>ing, transient<br>pain at site. | | Use after oral<br>hygiene, after<br>meals, and at<br>bedtime. | Used to treat<br>canker sores. |
| **Benzocaine**<br>Spec-T lozenge,<br>Orajel gel (OTC) | | Do not exceed<br>recommended<br>dosage. | | Used as an<br>anesthetic for<br>throat irritation. |
| **Benzocaine,<br>Cetylpyridinium<br>Chloride**<br>Cepacol Anesthetic<br>lozenge (OTC) | | Do not exceed<br>recommended<br>dosage. | | Used as an<br>anesthetic for<br>throat irritation<br>and as an<br>antiseptic. |
| **Benzocaine,<br>Orabase**<br>Orabase with<br>Benzocaine paste<br>(OTC) | | | | Used for relief<br>from mouth<br>sores. |
| **Carbamide<br>Peroxide**<br>Cankaid, Gly-Oxide<br>solution (OTC) | Inflammation,<br>irritation. | Do not use for<br>more than 7 days. | | Used for minor<br>inflammation of<br>gums and lips. |
| **Chlorhexidine<br>Gluconate**<br>Peridex oral<br>rinse (℞) | Staining of teeth;<br>altered taste<br>perception. | | Do not swallow;<br>expectorate after<br>rinsing. | Used to treat<br>gingivitis. |
| **Saliva<br>Substitutes**<br>Xero-Lube (OTC) | | | | Used for relief of<br>dry mouth and<br>throat in<br>xerostomia. |

**ACTION** Reduce inflammation in the mouth and throat.

**INDICATION** Generally for cold sores, fever blisters, irritation, and inflammation.

| Generic Name<br>*Brand Name* | Side Effects | Warnings | Dosing | Notes |
|---|---|---|---|---|
| **Tannic Acid**<br>*Zilactin Medicated*<br>gel (OTC) | Burning<br>sensation. | See a physician if<br>infection persists<br>for more than<br>10 days. | Wipe affected<br>area dry before<br>applying. | Used for relief<br>of pain and<br>burning from<br>cold sores and<br>fever blisters. |
| **Triamcinolone**<br>  **Acetate,**<br>  **Orabase**<br>*Kenalog in Orabase*<br>paste (℞) | | | | Used for treat-<br>ment of oral<br>lesions. |

## Nutritional Products

**ACTION** Vitamins and minerals are essential for normal metabolism. Vitamin deficiency can lead to certain diseases.

**INDICATION** Used to supplement the diet and to treat vitamin deficiencies. Most people on balanced diets do not need vitamin or mineral supplements.

| Generic Name<br>*Brand Name* | Side Effects | Warnings | Dosing | Notes |
|---|---|---|---|---|
| **Vitamin A**<br>*Aquasol A* drops,<br>tablet, capsule<br>(OTC) | Toxicity symp-<br>toms include nau-<br>sea, vomiting,<br>blurred vision,<br>bulging eyes,<br>tiredness, inflam-<br>mation of tongue<br>and lips, night<br>sweats. | Doses over<br>25,000 IU daily<br>should only be<br>taken with a<br>doctor's order. | | Fat-soluble vita-<br>min that pre-<br>vents night<br>blindness, pro-<br>motes growth,<br>and is essential<br>for healthy skin. |
| **Vitamin B₁**<br>*Thiamine* tablet<br>(OTC) | Nausea, weak-<br>ness, restless-<br>ness, shortness<br>of breath,<br>sweating. | | Oral thiamine has<br>been promoted<br>as a mosquito<br>repellant, how-<br>ever, effective-<br>ness has not<br>been proven. | Water-soluble<br>vitamin impor-<br>tant to carbo-<br>hydrate metabo-<br>lism in the body.<br>Thiamine defi-<br>ciency is known<br>as beriberi. |

Miscellaneous

**ACTION** Vitamins and minerals are essential for normal metabolism. Vitamin deficiency can lead to certain diseases.

**INDICATION** Used to supplement the diet and to treat vitamin deficiencies. Most people on balanced diets do not need vitamin or mineral supplements.

| Generic Name<br>*Brand Name* | Side Effects | Warnings | Dosing | Notes |
|---|---|---|---|---|
| **Vitamin B₂**<br>*Riboflavin* tablet<br>(OTC) | | | | Water-soluble vitamin important to metabolic functions in the body and to promote healthy skin and eyes. |
| **Vitamin B₃**<br>*Nicotinic Acid,*<br>*Niacin* tablet,<br>capsule, elixir<br>(OTC) | Nausea, vomiting, headache, flushing of face and neck, tingling skin, low blood pressure, restlessness. | | Take with food to avoid stomach upset. An aspirin 30 minutes before dose may reduce flushing effect. | Water-soluble vitamin used for niacin deficiency, pellagra, and to treat high cholesterol. |
| **Vitamin B₅**<br>*Pantothenic Acid,*<br>*Calcium Pantothenate* tablet<br>(OTC) | | | | Water-soluble vitamin used for pantothenic acid deficiency. |
| **Vitamin B₆**<br>*Pyridoxine* tablet<br>(OTC) | Numbness or tingling on skin, decreased touch, visual, and temperature sensation. | | | Water-soluble vitamin that acts in protein, carbohydrate, and fat metabolism. Used for pyridoxine deficiency. |
| **Vitamin C**<br>*Ascorbic Acid,*<br>*Sodium Ascorbate*<br>tablet, capsule,<br>powder, solution<br>(OTC) | Increased urination, kidney stones, diarrhea, mouth sores, nausea. | Use with caution in diabetes, history of kidney stones, and salt-restricted diets. | | Water-soluble vitamin used to prevent and treat scurvy and to acidify the urine. Used to promote healing for colds, infections, and general health; however, effectiveness has not been established. |

**ACTION** Vitamins and minerals are essential for normal metabolism. Vitamin deficiency can lead to certain diseases.

**INDICATION** Used to supplement the diet and to treat vitamin deficiencies. Most people on balanced diets do not need vitamin or mineral supplements.

| Generic Name<br>*Brand Name* | Side Effects | Warnings | Dosing | Notes |
|---|---|---|---|---|
| **Vitamin D**<br>*Calderol, Rocaltrol,*<br>*Vitamin D3,*<br>*Drisdol* tablet,<br>capsule (℞) | Loss of appetite, constipation, nausea, weakness, irritability, increased blood pressure. | Avoid mineral oil or magnesium-containing antacids. | Brands listed actually consist of various Vitamin D precursors and are not interchangeable. | Fat-soluble vitamin used to treat and prevent rickets (Vitamin D deficiency) and to regulate parathyroid hormone. Also used to treat certain types of calcium and phosphate disorders. |
| **Vitamin E**<br>*Aquasol E* drops,<br>tablet, capsule<br>(OTC) | Toxicity symptoms include nausea, diarrhea, tiredness, headache, blurred vision. | | | Fat-soluble vitamin that prevents "oxidation" reactions in the body. Used for Vitamin E deficiency, cancer, night leg cramps, heart disease, premenstrual problems, and to increase physical performance. |
| **Calcium**<br>*Calcium Gluconate,*<br>*Calcium Lactate,*<br>*Calcium Carbonate*<br>(OTC) | High calcium levels can cause loss of appetite, nausea, dry mouth, increased urination, constipation, and thirst. | Calcium can interfere with the absorption of other drugs. Allow at least 2 hours between calcium intake and other medications. | Vitamin D is often included in calcium products to increase the absorption of calcium from the digestive tract. | Mineral used to treat calcium deficiencies (osteoporosis, rickets), muscle cramps, and as a dietary supplement during pregnancy, breast feeding, and for childhood growth. |

Miscellaneous

**ACTION** Vitamins and minerals are essential for normal metabolism. Vitamin deficiency can lead to certain diseases.

**INDICATION** Used to supplement the diet and to treat vitamin deficiencies. Most people on balanced diets do not need vitamin or mineral supplements.

| Generic Name<br>Brand Name | Side Effects | Warnings | Dosing | Notes |
|---|---|---|---|---|
| **Fluoride**<br>*Sodium Fluoride, Stannous Fluoride, Luride* tablet,<br>rinse, drops,<br>gel (℞) | Toxicity symptoms include excess saliva, nausea, vomiting, tingling in fingers, muscle spasms, seizures, tooth staining. | | | Mineral used to control cavities and sometimes for osteoporosis. |
| **Iron**<br>*Ferrous Sulfate, Ferrous Gluconate, Ferrous Fumarate* tablet, capsule, liquid (OTC) | Constipation, diarrhea, black stools, GI irritation, nausea, staining of teeth. | | Take on an empty stomach. If GI upset occurs, take with food. | Used for the prevention and treatment of iron deficiency anemias. |
| **Magnesium**<br>*Magnesium Gluconate, Magnesium Carbonate* tablet<br>(OTC) | Diarrhea, nausea, abdominal cramps, fainting, dizziness. | Magnesium antacids may also be used as a dietary supplement. | | Electrolyte used to treat magnesium deficiency and sometimes to prevent recurrence of calcium oxalate kidney stones. |
| **Potassium**<br>*Potassium Chloride, Potassium Gluconate* tablet, capsule, liquid (℞) | Nausea, diarrhea, confusion, chest pain, shortness of breath, tingling of hands and feet. | | Take with meals to avoid stomach upset. Salt substitutes are another source of potassium. | Electrolyte used to treat hypokalemia (low potassium level) caused by low diet intake or increased excretion due to diarrhea, vomiting or other drugs (e.g., diuretics). |

**ACTION** Vitamins and minerals are essential for normal metabolism. Vitamin deficiency can lead to certain diseases.

**INDICATION** Used to supplement the diet and to treat vitamin deficiencies. Most people on balanced diets do not need vitamin or mineral supplements.

| Generic Name<br>*Brand Name* | Side Effects | Warnings | Dosing | Notes |
|---|---|---|---|---|
| **Zinc**<br>*Zinc Sulfate,*<br>*Zinc Gluconate*<br>  tablet, capsule<br>  (OTC) | Nausea, vomiting, dehydration, restlessness, diarrhea, ulcers. | | Take with food to avoid stomach upset. | Mineral used for zinc deficiency and sometimes used for delayed wound healing, acne, and other disorders. |

# Ophthalmic—Antibiotics

**ACTION** Stop infections by weakening bacterial cell walls, which results in the death of bacteria.

**INDICATION** Treatment of superficial eye infections.

**SIDE EFFECTS** Stinging, burning, irritation, allergic reaction, blurred vision, sensitivity to light, watering.

**WARNINGS/NOTES** Notify physician if burning or stinging becomes pronounced or pain persists.

| Generic Name | *Brand Name* |
|---|---|
| **Bacitracin** | *AK-Tracin* ointment (℞) |
| **Chloramphenicol** | *AK-Chlor* ointment (℞) |
| **Chloramphenicol** | *Chloroptic* solution, ointment (℞) |
| **Chlortetracycline** | *Aureomycin* ointment (℞) |
| **Ciprofloxacin** | *Ciloxan* solution (℞) |
| **Erythromycin** | *Ilotycin* ointment (℞) |
| **Gentamicin** | *Garamycin* solution, ointment (℞) |
| **Norfloxacin** | *Chibroxin* solution (℞) |
| **Ofloxacin** | *Ocuflox* solution (℞) |
| **Sodium Sulfacetamide** | *Sodium Sulamyd* solution (℞) |

Miscellaneous

**ACTION** Stop infections by weakening bacterial cell walls, which results in the death of bacteria.

**INDICATION** Treatment of superficial eye infections.

**SIDE EFFECTS** Stinging, burning, irritation, allergic reaction, blurred vision, sensitivity to light, watering.

**WARNINGS/NOTES** Notify physician if burning or stinging becomes pronounced or pain persists.

| Generic Name | Brand Name |
|---|---|
| **Sulfisoxazole** | *Gantrisin* ointment (℞) |
| **Tetracycline** | *Achromycin* suspension, ointment (℞) |
| **Tobramycin** | *Tobrex* solution, ointment (℞) |

## Ophthalmic—Antibiotic/Corticosteroid Combination

**ACTION** To treat bacterial infections and reduce inflammation in the eye.

**INDICATION** Treatment of eye inflammation along with infections.

**SIDE EFFECTS** Stinging, burning, blurred vision, sensitivity to light, irritation, headache.

**WARNINGS/NOTES** Long-term use may result in another bacterial or fungal infection requiring a change in drug therapy.

| Antibiotic Generic Name | Corticosteroid Generic Name | Brand Name |
|---|---|---|
| **Gentamicin** | **Prednisolone** | *Pred-G* suspension (℞) |
| **Neomycin** | **Dexamethasone** | *NeoDecadron* solution, ointment (℞) |
| **Neomycin, Polymyxin** | **Hydrocortisone** | *Cortisporin* suspension (℞) |
| **Neomycin, Polymyxin** | **Dexamethasone** | *Maxitrol* suspension, ointment (℞) |
| **Neomycin, Polymyxin** | **Dexamethasone** | *Dexacidin* suspension, ointment (℞) |
| **Sodium Sulfacetamide** | **Fluorometholone** | *FML-S* solution (℞) |
| **Sodium Sulfacetamide** | **Prednisolone** | *Blephamide* solution, ointment (℞) |

**ACTION** To treat bacterial infections and reduce inflammation in the eye.

**INDICATION** Treatment of eye inflammation along with infections.

**SIDE EFFECTS** Stinging, burning, blurred vision, sensitivity to light, irritation, headache.

**WARNINGS/NOTES** Long-term use may result in another bacterial or fungal infection requiring a change in drug therapy.

| Antibiotic Generic Name | Corticosteroid Generic Name | Brand Name |
|---|---|---|
| Sodium Sulfacetamide | Prednisolone | Vasocidin solution, ointment (℞) |
| Tobramycin | Dexamethasone | TobraDex suspension (℞) |

## Ophthalmic—Antiviral

**ACTION** Stop reproduction of viruses.

**INDICATION** Treatment of superficial viral eye infections.

**SIDE EFFECTS** Burning, stinging, pain, itching, allergic reactions, blurred vision, sensitivity to light.

**WARNINGS/NOTES** Recurrence may occur if therapy is not continued for 5 to 7 days after infection appears to be healed.

| Generic Name | Brand Name |
|---|---|
| Idoxuridine | Stoxil solution, ointment (℞) |
| Idoxuridine | Herplex solution (℞) |
| Trifluridine | Viroptic solution (℞) |
| Vidarabine | Vira-A ointment (℞) |

## Ophthalmic—Corticosteroid Agents

**ACTION** Corticosteroids inhibit the inflammatory response of the eye to mechanical, chemical, or allergy-causing agents.

**INDICATION** May be used for treatment of inflammation of the eye, injuries to corneas, certain eye surgeries, as well as other uses.

**SIDE EFFECTS** Blurring, stinging, burning, discomfort, pain, inflammation.

**WARNINGS/NOTES** May cause sensitivity to sunlight, which may be minimized by wearing sunglasses.

| Generic Name | Brand Name |
|---|---|
| Dexamethasone | *Maxidex* suspension, ointment (℞) |
| Dexamethasone | *Decadron Phosphate* solution, ointment (℞) |
| Fluorometholone | *Flarex* suspension (℞) |
| Fluorometholone | *Fluor-Op* suspension (℞) |
| Fluorometholone | *FML* suspension, ointment (℞) |
| Medrysone | *HMS* suspension (℞) |
| Prednisolone Acetate | *Econopred* suspension (℞) |
| Prednisolone Acetate | *Pred Forte* suspension (℞) |
| Prednisolone Acetate | *Pred Mild* suspension (℞) |
| Prednisolone Na Phosphate | *Inflamase Forte* solution (℞) |
| Prednisolone Na Phosphate | *Inflamase* solution (℞) |
| Rimexolone | *Vexol* solution (℞) |

# Ophthalmic—Glaucoma Agents

**ACTION** Reduction of intraocular fluid pressure by either decreasing the rate of production or increasing the outflow of fluid.

**INDICATION** Treatment of open-angle glaucoma or ocular hypertension.

**SIDE EFFECTS** Burning, stinging, tearing, blurred vision, dry eyes, light sensitivity, bitter taste following use.

**WARNINGS/NOTES** Generally wait at least 5 minutes before using other eye medications.

| Generic Name | Brand Name |
|---|---|
| **Apraclonidine HCl** | *Iopidine* solution (℞) |
| **Betaxolol HCl** | *Betoptic* solution (℞) |
| **Betaxolol HCl** | *Betoptic S* solution (℞) |
| **Brimonidine Tartrate** | *Alphagan* solution (℞) |
| **Carbachol** | *Isopto Carbachol* solution (℞) |
| **Carteolol** | *Ocupres* solution (℞) |
| **Demecarium Bromide** | *Humorsol* solution (℞) |
| **Dipivefrin HCl** | *Propine* solution (℞) |
| **Dorzolamide** | *Trusopt* solution (℞) |
| **Echothiophate Iodide** | *Phospholine Iodide* solution (℞) |
| **Epinephrine Borate** | *Epinal* solution (℞) |
| **Epinephrine, Pilocarpine** | *E-Pilo* solution (℞) |
| **Epinephrine HCl** | *Epifrin* solution (℞) |
| **Epinephrine HCl** | *Glaucon* solution (℞) |
| **Latanoprost** | *Xalatan* solution (℞) (Refrigerate) |
| **Levobunolol HCl** | *Betagen* solution (℞) |
| **Metipranolol HCl** | *OptiPranolol* solution (℞) |
| **Pilocarpine HCl** | *Isopto Carpine* solution (℞) |
| **Pilocarpine HCl** | *Pilocar* solution (℞) |
| **Pilocarpine HCl** | *Pilopine HS* gel (℞) |
| **Timolol Maleate** | *Timoptic* solution (℞) |
| **Timolol Maleate** | *Timoptic XE* solution (℞) |

## Ophthalmic—Mydriatic Agents

**ACTION** Relaxes the sphincter muscle of the iris, causing the pupil to dilate.

**INDICATION** Treatment of eye inflammation or for eye examinations.

**SIDE EFFECTS** Stinging, burning, blurred vision, sensitivity to light, irritation, headache.

**WARNINGS/NOTES** Avoid systemic absorption by pressing fingers on the corner of the eye next to the nose for 2 to 3 minutes after use.

| Generic Name | Brand Name |
|---|---|
| Atropine Sulfate | *Isopto Atropine* solution, ointment (℞) |
| Cyclopentolate | *Cyclogyl* solution (℞) |
| Homatropine HBr | *Isopto Homatropine* solution (℞) |
| Scopolamine HBr | *Isopto Hyoscine* solution (℞) |
| Tropicamide | *Mydriacyl* solution (℞) |

## Ophthalmic—NSAIDs

**ACTION** Nonsteroidal anti-inflammatory drugs (NSAIDs) inhibit the inflammatory response of the eye to mechanical, chemical, or allergy-causing agents.

**INDICATION** May be used for treatment of inflammation of the eye, injuries to corneas, certain eye surgeries, and other uses.

**SIDE EFFECTS** Blurring, stinging, burning, discomfort, pain, itching.

| Generic Name | Brand Name |
|---|---|
| Diclofenac Sodium | *Voltaren* solution (℞) |
| Flurbiprofen | *Ocufen* solution (℞) |
| Ketorolac | *Acular* solution (℞) |
| Suprofen | *Profenal* solution (℞) |

# Ophthalmic—Vasoconstrictor Agents

**ACTION** Reduce irritation and redness in the eye by causing vasoconstriction of conjunctival blood vessels.

**INDICATION** Treatment of irritations caused by smoke, smog, allergies, swimming, wind, or sun glare. Stronger formulations used for eye examinations.

**SIDE EFFECTS** Blurring, stinging, tearing, glaucoma, increased blood pressure, headache.

**WARNINGS/NOTES** Generally wait at least 5 minutes before using another eye medication.

| Generic Name | Brand Name |
|---|---|
| **Antazoline, Naphazoline** | *Vasocon-A* solution (OTC) |
| **Naphazoline** | *Vasocon* solution (℞) |
| **Naphazoline** | *VasoClear* solution (OTC) |
| **Naphazoline** | *Allerest* solution (OTC) |
| **Naphazoline** | *Naphcon* solution (OTC) |
| **Naphazoline** | *Naphcon Forte* solution (℞) |
| **Naphazoline, Pheniramine** | *Opcon-A* solution (OTC) |
| **Naphazoline, Pheniramine** | *Naphcon-A* solution (OTC) |
| **Oxymetazoline** | *Visine LR* solution (OTC) |
| **Phenylephrine** | *Mydrin* solution (℞) |
| **Phenylephrine** | *Prefin* solution (OTC) |
| **Tetrahydrozoline** | *Visine* solution (OTC) |
| **Tetrahydrozoline** | *Murine* solution (OTC) |

Miscellaneous

## Ophthalmic—Miscellaneous

**ACTION** Affects the eye directly.

**INDICATION** As noted.

| Generic Name<br>*Brand Name* | Side Effects | Warnings | Dosing | Notes |
|---|---|---|---|---|
| **Cromolyn Sodium**<br>*Opticrom* solution<br>(R) | Stinging, burning. | Do not wear soft contact lenses during use. | Must administer at regular intervals to work properly. | Used for treatment of allergic conjunctivitis. |
| **Natamycin**<br>*Natacyn* suspension (R) | | | Complete full regimen of therapy. | Used for fungal infections of the eye. |

## Oral—For Topical Purposes

**ACTION** These affect the skin.

**INDICATION** Used to treat various skin conditions.

| Generic Name<br>*Brand Name* | Side Effects | Warnings | Dosing | Notes |
|---|---|---|---|---|
| **Etretinate**<br>*Tegison* capsule (R) | Visual problems, stomachache, nausea, dizziness, chest pain, skin peeling. | Do not take vitamin A supplements. | Take with food, but not with milk. | Used to treat severe psoriasis. |
| **Isotretinoin**<br>*Accutane* capsule (R) | Headache, insomnia, visual disturbances, rash, dryness, nosebleed, weight loss. | Can cause fetal abnormalities; pregnancy must be avoided. | Take with meals. Avoid alcohol consumption. | Used to treat severe cystic acne. |
| **Methoxsalen**<br>*Oxsoralen* capsule (R) | Nausea, edema, leg cramps, itching. | Avoid sun exposure. | Take with food. | Used to treat severe psoriasis in conjunction with UV radiation. |

## Otics

**ACTION** Otics are preparations used in the ear.

**INDICATION** Otics are used against infections, to reduce inflammation and itching, to dissolve ear wax, and for pain relief. In general, keep head tilted or on side for at least 2 minutes after placing the drops. The earlobe should be held up and back in adults and down and back in children to assist penetration of the drops in the ear canal.

| Generic Name<br>*Brand Name* | Side Effects | Warnings | Dosing | Notes |
|---|---|---|---|---|
| **Acetic Acid**<br>*Domeboro, VoSol*<br>solution (℞) | Local irritation, itching, burning, redness, and rash. | | | Used to provide an acid medium and to provide antibacterial and antifungal actions. |
| **Acetic Acid,**<br>**Hydrocortisone**<br>*VoSol HC* solution<br>(℞) | Local irritation, itching, burning, redness, and rash. | | | Used to provide an acid medium, to provide antibacterial and antifungal actions, and for anti-inflammatory effect. |
| **Antipyrine,**<br>**Benzocaine**<br>*Auralgan* solution<br>(℞) | Local irritation, itching, burning, redness, and rash. | | | Used as a pain reliever. |
| **Boric Acid**<br>*Auro-Dri, Swim Ear*<br>solution (OTC) | Local irritation, itching, burning, redness, and rash. | | | Used to provide antibacterial and antifungal action. |
| **Carbamide**<br>  **Peroxide**<br>*Debrox, Murine Ear*<br>solution (OTC) | Local irritation, itching, burning, redness, and rash. | | | Used to dissolve ear wax. |
| **Hydrocortisone,**<br>  **Polymyxin**<br>*Otobiotic* solution<br>(℞) | Local irritation, itching, burning, redness, and rash. | | | Used to treat infection and inflammation. |

Miscellaneous

**ACTION** Otics are preparations used in the ear.

**INDICATION** Otics are used against infections, to reduce inflammation and itching, to dissolve ear wax, and for pain relief. In general, keep head tilted or on side for at least 2 minutes after placing the drops. The earlobe should be held up and back in adults and down and back in children to assist penetration of the drops in the ear canal.

| Generic Name<br>Brand Name | Side Effects | Warnings | Dosing | Notes |
|---|---|---|---|---|
| **Hydrocortisone, Neomycin, Polymyxin**<br>Cortisporin,<br>solution, suspension (℞) | Local irritation, itching, burning, redness, and rash. | | | Used to treat infection and inflammation. |
| **Triethanolamine**<br>Cerumenex<br>solution (℞) | Local irritation, itching, burning, redness, and rash. | | | Used to dissolve ear wax. |

## Rectal Products

**ACTION** Preparations containing anesthetics used to relieve pain, itching, and irritation. Hydrocortisone is used to reduce inflammation, itching, and swelling. Astringents shrink skin cells and lessen mucus and other secretions.

**INDICATION** These preparations are used for the anus and rectum to relieve the discomfort of hemorrhoids and itching or irritation. Many over-the-counter products contain ingredients that have not been demonstrated as effective. Not all ingredients are listed in the table. Dosage forms include suppository, cream, ointment, and aerosol foams.

**SIDE EFFECTS** Rash, itching, burning, redness, swelling.

**WARNINGS/NOTES** Maintain normal bowel movement with proper diet, exercise, and fluid intake. Do not use laxatives excessively. Stool softeners or bulk laxatives can be useful in assisting with the treatment.

| Corticosteroid | Anesthetic | Astringent | Brand Name |
|---|---|---|---|
| | **Benzocaine** | | Americaine (OTC) |
| | **Pramoxine** | **Zinc Oxide** | Anusol (OTC) |
| **Hydrocortisone Acetate** | | **Zinc Oxide** | Anusol HC (℞) |

**ACTION** Preparations containing anesthetics used to relieve pain, itching, and irritation. Hydrocortisone is used to reduce inflammation, itching, and swelling. Astringents shrink skin cells and lessen mucus and other secretions.

**INDICATION** These preparations are used for the anus and rectum to relieve the discomfort of hemorrhoids and itching or irritation. Many over-the-counter products contain ingredients that have not been demonstrated as effective. Not all ingredients are listed in the table. Dosage forms include suppository, cream, ointment, and aerosol foams.

**SIDE EFFECTS** Rash, itching, burning, redness, swelling.

**WARNINGS/NOTES** Maintain normal bowel movement with proper diet, exercise, and fluid intake. Do not use laxatives excessively. Stool softeners or bulk laxatives can be useful in assisting with the treatment.

| Corticosteroid | Anesthetic | Astringent | Brand Name |
|---|---|---|---|
| Hydrocortisone Acetate | Dibucaine | | Corticaine (℞) |
| Hydrocortisone | | | Proctocort (℞) |
| | Pramoxine | | Proctofoam (OTC) |
| Hydrocortisone Acetate | Pramoxine | | Proctofoam-HC (℞) |
| | | Witch Hazel | Tucks Pads (OTC) |
| | Pramoxine | Zinc Oxide | Tronolane (OTC) |

## Smoking Cessation Products

**ACTION** Reduce craving and other effects of nicotine withdrawal.

**INDICATION** To assist in stop smoking. Treatment is more effective when combined with a smoking cessation program.

| Generic Name Brand Name | Side Effects | Warnings | Dosing | Notes |
|---|---|---|---|---|
| **Bupropion HCL** Zyban sustained-release tablet (℞) | Dry mouth, insomnia, dizziness, nausea, vomiting. | Avoid alcohol and other depressants. | | |
| **Nicotine** Habitrol, Nicoderm, Nicotrol topical patch (OTC, ℞) | Burning, itching, increased cough, nausea, sleepiness, insomnia. | Stop smoking completely. | | |

**ACTION** Reduce craving and other effects of nicotine withdrawal.

**INDICATION** To assist in stop smoking. Treatment is more effective when combined with a smoking cessation program.

| Generic Name<br>*Brand Name* | Side Effects | Warnings | Dosing | Notes |
|---|---|---|---|---|
| **Nicotine**<br>**Polacrilex**<br>*Nicorette* gum<br>(OTC) | Jaw ache, hic-coughs, nausea, vomiting, eruc-tation, excess salivation. | Do not continue to smoke while using gum therapy. | Do not exceed 30 pieces of gum a day. | |

## Topical—Acne Products

**ACTION** These products work either by antibacterial action against bacteria in the pores of the skin, or by removal of excess sebum, or by drying action.

**INDICATION** Used to treat various types of acne.

| Generic Name<br>*Brand Name* | Side Effects | Warnings | Dosing | Notes |
|---|---|---|---|---|
| **Adapalene**<br>*Differin* gel (℞) | Erythema, scaling, dryness, pruritus. | Avoid contact with eyes. May make sensitive to sunlight and sunlamps. | | |
| **Azelaic Acid**<br>*Azelex* cream (℞) | Itching, rash, stinging, tingling, irritation, red-ness, dryness. | Avoid contact with eyes. | Wash skin thoroughly and dry before apply-ing a thin layer. | |
| **Benzoyl Peroxide**<br>*Benzac W, Oxy-10, Fostex, Clearasil, Desquam* cleanser, lotion, cream, gel<br>(OTC or ℞) | Itching, stinging, tingling, rash, irritation, red-ness, dryness. | Avoid contact with eyes. | Wash skin thoroughly and dry before apply-ing a thin layer. | May bleach hair or colored fabric. |
| **Tazarotene**<br>*Tazorac* gel (℞) | Burning, sting-ing, dry skin, erythema. | Avoid exposure to sunlamps and excessive sunlight. | | May be used to treat psoriasis. |

**ACTION** These products work either by antibacterial action against bacteria in the pores of the skin, or by removal of excess sebum, or by drying action.

**INDICATION** Used to treat various types of acne.

| Generic Name<br>*Brand Name* | Side Effects | Warnings | Dosing | Notes |
|---|---|---|---|---|
| **Tretinoin**<br>*Retin-A* cream, gel, liquid (℞)<br>*Retin-A Micro* gel (℞) | Itching, stinging, tingling, rash, irritation, redness, dryness. | Avoid contact with eyes. May make sensitive to sunlight. | Wash skin thoroughly and dry before applying a thin layer. | Unapproved use as a wrinkle remover. |

## Topical—Anesthetics

**ACTION** Inhibit conduction of nerve impulses from sensory nerves.

**INDICATION** To relieve pain at local application.

**SIDE EFFECTS** Burning, tenderness, tissue irritation, swelling.

**WARNINGS/NOTES** If using medications for the mouth, avoid food and gum for 1 hour after treatment.

| Generic Name | *Brand Name* |
|---|---|
| **Dibucaine** | *Nupercainal* cream, ointment (OTC) |
| **Lidocaine** | *Xylocaine* ointment (OTC) |
| **Lidocaine** | *Xylocaine Viscous* oral solution (℞) |
| **Benzocaine** | *Americaine* solution (OTC) |
| **Benzocaine** | *Dermoplast* solution (OTC) |
| **Butamben Picrate** | *Butesin Picrate* ointment (OTC) |
| **Tetracaine** | *Pontocaine* ointment (OTC) |
| **Pramoxine HCl** | *Tronothane* cream (OTC) |

## Topical—Antibiotics

**ACTION** Antibiotics kill bacteria by preventing the formation of the normal cell bacterial wall, thereby increasing the likelihood that the cell will rupture.

**INDICATION** Used to treat skin infections caused by bacteria. It is important to take the full course of therapy to prevent a reoccurrence of the infection. Many are used for acne.

| Generic Name<br>*Brand Name* | Side Effects | Warnings | Dosing | Notes |
|---|---|---|---|---|
| **Bacitracin**<br>*Baciguent* topical ointment (OTC) | Rash, itching, burning, redness, swelling. | Avoid contact with eyes. | Use a thin layer. May cover with loose gauze dressing. | Used to treat superficial skin infection or to prevent infections of minor cuts and scrapes. |
| **Chloramphenicol**<br>*Chloromycetin* topical cream (℞) | Rash, itching, burning, redness, swelling. | Avoid contact with eyes. | Use a thin layer. May cover with loose gauze dressing. | Used to treat superficial skin infection or to prevent infections of minor cuts and scrapes. |
| **Chlortetracycline**<br>*Aureomycin* topical ointment (℞) | Skin irritation, burning, rash, itching, yellow staining of skin. | Avoid contact with eyes and lining of the nose and mouth. | | Used to treat acne vulgaris and to treat superficial skin infections. |
| **Clindamycin**<br>*Cleocin T, C/T/S, Clinda-Derm* gel, lotion, topical solution (℞) | Rash, hives, itching, redness, dryness, flaking, peeling, burning, or oily skin. | Avoid contact with eyes, nose, mouth, and other mucous membranes and damaged skin. This may result in burning or irritation. | Clean and dry skin before applying. | Used to treat acne. |
| **Erythromycin**<br>*Staticin, A/T/S, Eryderm, Erycette* topical solution (℞)<br>*A/T/S, Erygel* topical gel (℞)<br>*Akne-Mycin* ointment (℞) | Redness, flushing, sloughing, dryness, itching, oily skin. | Avoid contact with eyes, nose, mouth, and other mucous membranes and damaged skin. | Clean and dry skin before applying. | Used to treat acne vulgaris. |

**ACTION** Antibiotics kill bacteria by preventing the formation of the normal cell bacterial wall, thereby increasing the likelihood that the cell will rupture.

**INDICATION** Used to treat skin infections caused by bacteria. It is important to take the full course of therapy to prevent a reoccurrence of the infection. Many are used for acne.

| Generic Name<br>*Brand Name* | Side Effects | Warnings | Dosing | Notes |
|---|---|---|---|---|
| **Erythromycin, Benzoyl Peroxide** *Benzamycin* topical gel (℞) | Redness, flushing, sloughing, dryness, itching, oily skin. | Avoid contact with eyes, nose, mouth, and other mucous membranes and damaged skin. | Clean and dry skin before applying. | Used to treat acne vulgaris. Store in refrigerator. Unused drug should be discarded after 3 months. |
| **Gentamicin** *Garamycin* topical ointment (℞) | Rash, itching, burning, redness, swelling. | Avoid contact with eyes. May make sensitive to sunlight. | Use a thin layer. May cover with loose gauze dressing. | Used to treat superficial skin infection or to prevent infections of minor cuts and scrapes. |
| **Meclocycline Sulfosalicylate** *Meclan* topical cream (℞) | Skin irritation, burning, rash, itching, yellow staining of skin. | Avoid contact with eyes, and lining of the nose and mouth. | | Used to treat acne vulgaris and to treat superficial skin infection. |
| **Metronidazole** *MetroGel* topical gel (℞) | Redness, mild dryness, burning, and irritation of the skin. | Avoid contact with eyes. | Wash area before application. | Used to treat inflammatory papules and pustules and acne rosacea. |
| **Mupirocin** *Bactroban* topical cream or ointment (℞) *Bactroban* nasal ointment (℞) | Burning, stinging, pain, itching, rash, dry skin, redness, swelling. | Do not use near or in eyes. | A loose gauze dressing may be used to cover area. | Used to treat impetigo. |
| **Neomycin Sulfate** *Myciguent* topical cream or ointment (OTC) | Rash, itching, burning, redness, swelling. | Avoid contact with eyes. | Use a thin layer. May cover with loose gauze dressing. | Used to treat superficial skin infection or to prevent infections of minor cuts and scrapes. |

**ACTION** Antibiotics kill bacteria by preventing the formation of the normal cell bacterial wall, thereby increasing the likelihood that the cell will rupture.

**INDICATION** Used to treat skin infections caused by bacteria. It is important to take the full course of therapy to prevent a reoccurrence of the infection. Many are used for acne.

| Generic Name<br>Brand Name | Side Effects | Warnings | Dosing | Notes |
|---|---|---|---|---|
| **Oxytetracycline, Polymyxin B Sulfate**<br>Terramycin with Polymyxin ointment (OTC) | Rash, itching, burning, redness, swelling. | Avoid contact with eyes. | Use a thin layer. May cover with loose gauze dressing. | Used to treat superficial skin infection or to prevent infections of minor cuts and scrapes. |
| **Polymyxin B Sulfate, Neomycin Base**<br>Neosporin cream (OTC) | Rash, itching, burning, redness, swelling. | Avoid contact with eyes. | Use a thin layer. May cover with loose gauze dressing. | Used to treat superficial skin infection or to prevent infections of minor cuts and scrapes. |
| **Polymyxin B Sulfate, Neomycin Base, Bacitracin**<br>Triple Antibiotic, Mycitracin, Neosporin topical ointment (OTC) | Rash, itching, burning, redness, swelling. | Avoid contact with eyes. | Use a thin layer. May cover with loose gauze dressing. | Used to treat superficial skin infection or to prevent infections of minor cuts and scrapes. |
| **Polymyxin B Sulfate, Zinc Bacitracin**<br>Polysporin ointment, powder, aerosol (OTC) | Rash, itching, burning, redness, swelling. | Avoid contact with eyes. | Use a thin layer. May cover with loose gauze dressing. | Used to treat superficial skin infection or to prevent infections of minor cuts and scrapes. |
| **Tetracycline**<br>Topicycline topical solution (℞) | Skin irritation, burning, rash, itching, yellow staining of skin. | Avoid contact with eyes and lining of the nose and mouth. | | Used to treat acne vulgaris and superficial skin infection. |

# Topical—Antifungals

**ACTION** Antifungals typically interfere with the formation of the cell membrane of the fungi. This results in leakage of cellular contents and death of the fungi cell.

**INDICATION** Used to treat various fungal infections such as athlete's foot, jock itch, ringworm, Tinea versicolor, candidiasis (yeast), and eczema. It is important to use the full course of therapy to prevent a recurrence of the infection.

| Generic Name<br>*Brand Name* | Side Effects | Warnings | Dosing | Notes |
|---|---|---|---|---|
| **Amphotericin B**<br>*Fungizone* cream, lotion, ointment (℞) | Drying, skin discoloration, redness, itching, burning, rash. | May cause staining of fabrics. | Apply liberally to clean affected areas. | Used for Candida infections. |
| **Butenafine HCl**<br>*Mentax* cream (℞) | Contact dermatitis, erythema, irritation, itching. | Avoid contact with the eyes and other mucous membranes. | Wash hands after applying. Do not use occlusive dressings. | Used for athlete's foot, ringworm, and groin fungus. |
| **Ciclopirox Olamine**<br>*Loprox* cream, lotion (℞) | Irritation, burning, redness. | Do not use occlusive wrappings or dressings. | Clean and dry skin before applying. Continue treatment for complete course of therapy. | |
| **Clioquinol (Iodochlorhydroxyquin)**<br>*Vioform* cream, ointment (OTC) | Itching, redness, swelling, pain, irritation. | Not to be used for more than 1 week. | May stain fabric, hair, and skin. | Used for eczema, athlete's foot and other fungal infections. |
| **Clotrimazole**<br>*Lotrimin AF, Mycelex* OTC cream, solution<br>*Lotrimin* lotion (℞, OTC) | Erythema, stinging, edema, blistering, pruritus. | Keep out of eyes. | Clean area before applying. | |
| **Econazole Nitrate**<br>*Spectazole* cream (℞) | Erythema, stinging, itching. | Keep out of eyes. | Clean and dry skin before applying. Complete therapy even if symptoms clear up. | |

**ACTION** Antifungals typically interfere with the formation of the cell membrane of the fungi. This results in leakage of cellular contents and death of the fungi cell.

**INDICATION** Used to treat various fungal infections such as athlete's foot, jock itch, ringworm, Tinea versicolor, candidiasis (yeast), and eczema. It is important to use the full course of therapy to prevent a recurrence of the infection.

| Generic Name<br>*Brand Name* | Side Effects | Warnings | Dosing | Notes |
|---|---|---|---|---|
| **Gentian Violet**<br>*Gentian Violet*<br>solution (OTC) | | Will stain cloth-ing and skin. Do not apply to ulcerative lesions. | | |
| **Haloprogin**<br>*Halotex* cream,<br>solution (℞) | Burning sensa-tion, scaling, erythema. | Keep out of eyes. | | |
| **Ketoconazole**<br>*Nizoral* cream,<br>shampoo (℞) | Irritation, pru-ritus, stinging. | | | |
| **Miconazole Nitrate**<br>*Micatin,*<br>*Monistat-Derm*<br>cream, powder<br>(OTC) | Burning, itching, stinging, itching. | If no improve-ment after 2 to 4 weeks, notify physician. | Although symp-toms may be re-lieved in 2 to 3 days, treatment should be com-pleted to avoid recurrence. | Used for athlete's foot and Tinea versicolor. |
| **Naftifine HCl**<br>*Naftin* cream,<br>gel (℞) | Burning, stinging, dryness, itching. | Avoid occlusive dressings and wraps. Keep away from eyes, nose, and other mucous mem-branes. | Wash hands after applying medication. | |
| **Nystatin**<br>*Mycostatin, Nilstat*<br>cream, ointment<br>(℞) | | | Apply after cleaning area. | Used for Candida infections. |
| **Oxiconazole Nitrate**<br>*Oxistat* cream,<br>lotion (℞) | Itching, burning, irritation, ery-thema, fissuring. | Keep out of eyes. | Apply in the evening. | |

**ACTION** Antifungals typically interfere with the formation of the cell membrane of the fungi. This results in leakage of cellular contents and death of the fungi cell.

**INDICATION** Used to treat various fungal infections such as athlete's foot, jock itch, ringworm, Tinea versicolor, candidiasis (yeast), and eczema. It is important to use the full course of therapy to prevent a recurrence of the infection.

| Generic Name<br>*Brand Name* | Side Effects | Warnings | Dosing | Notes |
|---|---|---|---|---|
| **Sulconazole Nitrate**<br>*Exelderm* cream, solution (℞) | Itching, burning, stinging. | Keep out of eyes. | Complete therapy to avoid a recurrence. | |
| **Terbinafine HCl**<br>*Lamisil* cream (℞) | | | | |
| **Tolnaftate**<br>*Tinactin, NP-27* cream, solution, powder, spray (OTC) | Mild irritation. | Not for nail or scalp infections. | Clean and dry skin before applying. Discontinue if symptoms do not improve in 10 days. | |
| **Triacetin**<br>*Fungoid* solution, cream (OTC) | Itching, irritation. | Cover with bandages to avoid contact with rayon fabrics. | Clean skin with alcohol or soap and water before applying. Use for 1 week after symptoms disappear. | Used for athlete's foot and superficial fungal infections. |
| **Undecylenic Acid**<br>*Cruex, Desenex* powder, ointment, cream (OTC) | Burning, irritation, rash, stinging. | Avoid inhaling and contact with eyes and mucus membranes. Do not apply to raw skin or deep wounds. | Cleanse and dry area well before applying. | Used for athlete's foot, ringworm, jock itch, diaper rash, prickly heat. |

## Topical—Antivirals

**ACTION** Interfere with replication of virus.

**INDICATION** Used to treat various topical viral infections.

| Generic Name<br>*Brand Name* | Side Effects | Warnings | Dosing | Notes |
|---|---|---|---|---|
| **Acyclovir**<br>*Zovirax* ointment<br>(℞) | Burning, stinging, itching. | Avoid use in or near the eyes. | Use rubber gloves or finger cots when applying ointment to reduce the risk of spreading the infection. | Avoid sexual intercourse when sores are present to prevent infecting sex partner. |
| **Penciclovir**<br>*Denavir* cream (℞) | Headache. | Avoid use near the eyes. | Use rubber gloves or finger cots when applying ointment to reduce the risk of spreading the infection. | |

## Topical—Corticosteroids

**ACTION** Topical corticosteroids have anti-inflammatory, antipruritic, and vasoconstrictive activities dependent on the extent of absorption and the potency of the product.

**INDICATION** Use is indicated for numerous skin disorders that are responsive to corticosteroids. This includes, but is not limited to, contact dermatitis, eczema, psoriasis, insect bites, poison ivy, allergic rashes, and general itching.

**BANNED SUBSTANCES** NCAA and/or USOC may list some of these substances as banned for athletes to use.

| Generic Name<br>*Brand Name* | Side Effects | Warnings | Dosing | Notes |
|---|---|---|---|---|
| **Alclometasone Dipropionate**<br>*Aclovate* cream, ointment (℞) | Burning, itching, irritation, skin atrophy. | Avoid prolonged use and use in the eyes. | Apply sparingly as a thin film and rub in lightly. Wash area before applying. | Used to treat skin inflammation and itching. |

**ACTION** Topical corticosteroids have anti-inflammatory, antipruritic, and vasoconstrictive activities dependent on the extent of absorption and the potency of the product.

**INDICATION** Use is indicated for numerous skin disorders that are responsive to corticosteroids. This includes, but is not limited to, contact dermatitis, eczema, psoriasis, insect bites, poison ivy, allergic rashes, and general itching.

**BANNED SUBSTANCES** NCAA and/or USOC may list some of these substances as banned for athletes to use.

| Generic Name *Brand Name* | Side Effects | Warnings | Dosing | Notes |
|---|---|---|---|---|
| **Amcinonide** *Cylocort* cream, ointment, lotion (℞) | Burning, itching, irritation, skin atrophy. | Avoid prolonged use and use in the eyes. | Apply sparingly as a thin film and rub in lightly. Wash area before applying. | Used to treat skin inflammation and itching. |
| **Betamethasone** *Uticort* cream, lotion, gel (℞) | Burning, itching, irritation, skin atrophy. | Avoid prolonged use and use in the eyes. | Apply sparingly as a thin film and rub in lightly. Wash area before applying. | Used to treat skin inflammation and itching. |
| **Betamethasone Dipropionate** *Diprolene, Diprosone* cream, ointment, lotion, aerosol (℞) | Burning, itching, irritation, skin atrophy. | Avoid prolonged use and use in the eyes. | Apply sparingly as a thin film and rub in lightly. Wash area before applying. | Used to treat skin inflammation and itching. |
| **Betamethasone Valerate** *Valisone* cream, ointment, lotion (℞) | Burning, itching, irritation, skin atrophy. | Avoid prolonged use and use in the eyes. | Apply sparingly as a thin film and rub in lightly. Wash area before applying. | Used to treat skin inflammation and itching. |
| **Clobetasol Propionate** *Temovate* cream, ointment (℞) | Burning, itching, irritation, skin atrophy. | Avoid prolonged use and use in the eyes. | Apply sparingly as a thin film and rub in lightly. Wash area before applying. | Used to treat skin inflammation and itching. |
| **Clocortolone Pivalate** *Cloderm* cream (℞) | Burning, itching, irritation, skin atrophy. | Avoid prolonged use and use in the eyes. | Apply sparingly as a thin film and rub in lightly. Wash area before applying. | Used to treat skin inflammation and itching. |

Miscellaneous

**ACTION** Topical corticosteroids have anti-inflammatory, antipruritic, and vasoconstrictive activities dependent on the extent of absorption and the potency of the product.

**INDICATION** Use is indicated for numerous skin disorders that are responsive to corticosteroids. This includes, but is not limited to, contact dermatitis, eczema, psoriasis, insect bites, poison ivy, allergic rashes, and general itching.

**BANNED SUBSTANCES** NCAA and/or USOC may list some of these substances as banned for athletes to use.

| Generic Name<br>*Brand Name* | Side Effects | Warnings | Dosing | Notes |
|---|---|---|---|---|
| **Desonide**<br>*DesOwen,*<br>*Tridesilon* cream,<br>ointment (℞) | Burning, itching,<br>irritation, skin<br>atrophy. | Avoid prolonged<br>use and use in<br>the eyes. | Apply sparingly<br>as a thin film and<br>rub in lightly.<br>Wash area be-<br>fore applying. | Used to treat<br>skin inflamma-<br>tion and itching. |
| **Desoximetasone**<br>*Topicort, Topicort LP*<br>cream, ointment,<br>gel (℞) | Burning, itching,<br>irritation, skin<br>atrophy. | Avoid prolonged<br>use and use in<br>the eyes. | Apply sparingly<br>as a thin film and<br>rub in lightly.<br>Wash area be-<br>fore applying. | Used to treat<br>skin inflamma-<br>tion and itching. |
| **Dexamethasone**<br>*Decaderm,*<br>*Decadron, Deca-*<br>*spray* cream, gel,<br>aerosol (℞) | Burning, itching,<br>irritation, skin<br>atrophy. | Avoid prolonged<br>use and use in<br>the eyes. | Apply sparingly<br>as a thin film and<br>rub in lightly.<br>Wash area be-<br>fore applying. | Used to treat<br>skin inflamma-<br>tion and itching. |
| **Diflorasone**<br>**Diacetate**<br>*Florone, Psorcon*<br>cream, ointment<br>(℞) | Burning, itching,<br>irritation, skin<br>atrophy. | Avoid prolonged<br>use and use in<br>the eyes. | Apply sparingly<br>as a thin film and<br>rub in lightly.<br>Wash area be-<br>fore applying. | Used to treat<br>skin inflamma-<br>tion and itching. |
| **Fluocinolone**<br>**Acetonide**<br>*Synalar, Fluonid*<br>cream, ointment<br>solution (℞) | Burning, itching,<br>irritation, skin<br>atrophy. | Avoid prolonged<br>use and use in<br>the eyes. | Apply sparingly<br>as a thin film and<br>rub in lightly.<br>Wash area be-<br>fore applying. | Used to treat<br>skin inflamma-<br>tion and itching. |
| **Fluocinonide**<br>*Lidex, Lidex-E* cream,<br>*Synalar, Fluonid*<br>ointment, solu-<br>tion gel (℞) | Burning, itching,<br>irritation, skin<br>atrophy. | Avoid prolonged<br>use and use in<br>the eyes. | Apply sparingly<br>as a thin film and<br>rub in lightly.<br>Wash area be-<br>fore applying. | Used to treat<br>skin inflamma-<br>tion and itching. |

**ACTION** Topical corticosteroids have anti-inflammatory, antipruritic, and vasoconstrictive activities dependent on the extent of absorption and the potency of the product.

**INDICATION** Use is indicated for numerous skin disorders that are responsive to corticosteroids. This includes, but is not limited to, contact dermatitis, eczema, psoriasis, insect bites, poison ivy, allergic rashes, and general itching.

**BANNED SUBSTANCES** NCAA and/or USOC may list some of these substances as banned for athletes to use.

| Generic Name<br>*Brand Name* | Side Effects | Warnings | Dosing | Notes |
|---|---|---|---|---|
| **Flurandrenolide**<br>*Cordran* cream,<br>ointment, lotion,<br>tape (℞) | Burning, itching,<br>irritation, skin<br>atrophy. | Avoid prolonged<br>use and use in<br>the eyes. | Apply sparingly<br>as a thin film and<br>rub in lightly.<br>Wash area be-<br>fore applying. | Used to treat<br>skin inflamma-<br>tion and itching. |
| **Fluticasone<br>Propionate**<br>*Cutivate* cream,<br>ointment (℞) | Burning, itching,<br>irritation, skin<br>atrophy. | Avoid prolonged<br>use and use in<br>the eyes. | Apply sparingly<br>as a thin film and<br>rub in lightly.<br>Wash area be-<br>fore applying. | Used to treat<br>skin inflamma-<br>tion and itching. |
| **Halcinonide<br>Propionate**<br>*Halog* cream,<br>ointment solution<br>(℞) | Burning, itching,<br>irritation, skin<br>atrophy. | Avoid prolonged<br>use and use in<br>the eyes. | Apply sparingly<br>as a thin film and<br>rub in lightly.<br>Wash area be-<br>fore applying. | Used to treat<br>skin inflamma-<br>tion and itching. |
| **Halobetasol<br>Propionate**<br>*Ultravate* cream,<br>ointment (℞) | Burning, itching,<br>irritation, skin<br>atrophy. | Avoid prolonged<br>use and use in<br>the eyes. | Apply sparingly<br>as a thin film and<br>rub in lightly.<br>Wash area be-<br>fore applying. | Used to treat<br>skin inflamma-<br>tion and itching. |
| **Hydrocortisone**<br>*Cortizone, Cortaid,<br>Hytone* cream,<br>ointment, lotion<br>(OTC, ℞) | Burning, itching,<br>irritation, skin<br>atrophy. | Avoid prolonged<br>use and use in<br>the eyes. | Apply sparingly<br>as a thin film and<br>rub in lightly.<br>Wash area be-<br>fore applying. | Used to treat<br>skin inflamma-<br>tion and itching. |
| **Hydrocortisone<br>Buteprate**<br>*Pandel* cream,<br>ointment (℞) | Burning, itching,<br>irritation, skin<br>atrophy. | Avoid prolonged<br>use and use in<br>the eyes. | Apply sparingly<br>as a thin film and<br>rub in lightly.<br>Wash area be-<br>fore applying. | Used to treat<br>skin inflamma-<br>tion and itching. |

Miscellaneous

**ACTION** Topical corticosteroids have anti-inflammatory, antipruritic, and vasoconstrictive activities dependent on the extent of absorption and the potency of the product.

**INDICATION** Use is indicated for numerous skin disorders that are responsive to corticosteroids. This includes, but is not limited to, contact dermatitis, eczema, psoriasis, insect bites, poison ivy, allergic rashes, and general itching.

**BANNED SUBSTANCES** NCAA and/or USOC may list some of these substances as banned for athletes to use.

| Generic Name<br>*Brand Name* | Side Effects | Warnings | Dosing | Notes |
|---|---|---|---|---|
| **Hydrocortisone Butyrate** <br>*Locoid* cream, ointment (℞) | Burning, itching, irritation, skin atrophy. | Avoid prolonged use and use in the eyes. | Apply sparingly as a thin film and rub in lightly. Wash area before applying. | Used to treat skin inflammation and itching. |
| **Hydrocortisone Valerate** <br>*Westcort* cream, ointment (℞) | Burning, itching, irritation, skin atrophy. | Avoid prolonged use and use in the eyes. | Apply sparingly as a thin film and rub in lightly. Wash area before applying. | Used to treat skin inflammation and itching. |
| **Mometasone Furoate** <br>*Elocon* cream, ointment, lotion (℞) | Burning, itching, irritation, skin atrophy. | Avoid prolonged use and use in the eyes. | Apply sparingly as a thin film and rub in lightly. Wash area before applying. | Used to treat skin inflammation and itching. |
| **Triamcinolone Acetonide** <br>*Aristocort, Kenalog* cream, ointment, lotion (℞) | Burning, itching, irritation, skin atrophy. | Avoid prolonged use and use in the eyes. | Apply sparingly as a thin film and rub in lightly. Wash area before applying. | Used to treat skin inflammation and itching. |

# Topical—Corticosteroid/Antibiotic Combinations

Consult individual ingredient products for more information.

| Corticosteroid | Antibiotic | Brand Name |
|---|---|---|
| **Hydrocortisone** | **Neomycin Sulfate** | Neo-Cortef cream, ointment (℞) |
| **Fluocinolone Acetonide** | **Neomycin Sulfate** | Neo-Synalar cream (℞) |
| **Flurandrenolide** | **Neomycin Sulfate** | Cordran-N cream, ointment (℞) |
| **Dexamethasone** | **Neomycin Sulfate** | NeoDecadron cream (℞) |
| **Hydrocortisone** | **Bacitracin, Polymyxin B, Neomycin Sulfate** | Cortisporin ointment (℞) |

# Topical—Corticosteroid/Antifungal Combinations

Consult individual ingredient products for more information.

| Corticosteroid | Antifungal | Brand Name |
|---|---|---|
| **Betamethasone** | **Clotrimazole** | Lotrisone cream (℞) |
| **Triamcinolone Acetonide** | **Nystatin** | Mycolog-II cream, ointment (℞) |
| **Triamcinolone Acetonide** | **Nystatin** | Mytrex cream, ointment (℞) |

# Topical—Rubs and Liniments

**ACTION** Reduce inflammation and pain.

**INDICATION** For the relief of pain of muscular aches, neuralgia, rheumatism, sprains, and other conditions when the skin is intact.

**SIDE EFFECTS** Local irritation. Salicylate products may cause tinnitus, nausea, and vomiting.

**WARNINGS/NOTES** Consult a physician if pain persists for more than 7 days.

| Generic Name | Brand Name |
|---|---|
| **Menthol, Acetone, Chloroxylenol** | Absorbine Jr. liniment (OTC) |
| **Methyl Salicylate, Menthol** | Ben-Gay balm, ointment, gel (OTC) |

Miscellaneous

**ACTION** Reduce inflammation and pain.

**INDICATION** For the relief of pain of muscular aches, neuralgia, rheumatism, sprains, and other conditions when the skin is intact.

**SIDE EFFECTS** Local irritation. Salicylate products may cause tinnitus, nausea, and vomiting.

**WARNINGS/NOTES** Consult a physician if pain persists for more than 7 days.

| Generic Name | Brand Name |
|---|---|
| **Methyl Salicylate, Menthol** | *Icy Hot* balm (OTC) |
| **Triethanolamine Salicylate** | *Mobisyl* cream (OTC) |
| **Triethanolamine Salicylate** | *Myoflex* cream (OTC) |
| **Triethanolamine Salicylate** | *Aspercreme* (OTC) |

## Topical—Pediculicides

**ACTION** These anti-infectives kill selected organisms.

**INDICATION** Used for treatment of various organisms such as lice and scabies.

| Generic Name<br>Brand Name | Side Effects | Warnings | Dosing | Notes |
|---|---|---|---|---|
| **Crotamiton**<br>*Eurax* cream,<br>lotion (℞) | Allergic skin irritation, burning, itching, stinging, redness, swelling, rash. | Avoid contact with eyes, open cuts, mouth, and nose. | Wash clothing and bed linens following application. | Used to treat scabies. |
| **Lindane**<br>*Kwell, Scabene*<br>cream, lotion,<br>shampoo (℞) | Allergic skin irritation, burning, itching, stinging, redness, swelling, rash. | Avoid contact with eyes, open cuts, mouth, and nose. | Wash clothing and bed linens following application. | Used to treat scabies and lice. |
| **Permethrin**<br>*Nix* lotion (OTC)<br>cream (℞) | Allergic skin irritation, burning, itching, stinging, redness, swelling, rash. | Avoid contact with eyes, open cuts, mouth, and nose. | Wash clothing and bed linens following application. | Used to treat lice. |

**ACTION** These anti-infectives kill selected organisms.

**INDICATION** Used for treatment of various organisms such as lice and scabies.

| Generic Name<br>*Brand Name* | Side Effects | Warnings | Dosing | Notes |
|---|---|---|---|---|
| **Pyrethrins**<br>*RID, R&C, A-200* gel,<br>liquid, shampoo<br>(OTC) | Avoid contact<br>with eyes, open<br>cuts, mouth, and<br>nose. | Allergic skin irri-<br>tation, burning,<br>itching, stinging,<br>redness, swell-<br>ing, rash. | Wash clothing<br>and bed linens<br>following appli-<br>cation. | Used to treat<br>lice. |

## Topical—Miscellaneous

**ACTION** These products work by a variety of mechanism to affect skin coloring, tone, elasticity, pain, dryness, and removal of dead skin.

**INDICATION** These products are used for dandruff, psoriasis, seborrhea, and burns, and as anesthetics, analgesics, antihistamines, antiseptics, and liniments.

| Generic Name<br>*Brand Name* | Side Effects | Warnings | Dosing | Notes |
|---|---|---|---|---|
| **Anthralin**<br>*Anthra-Derm,*<br>*Drithocreme*<br>ointment, cream<br>(℞) | Irritation, dis-<br>coloration of<br>fingernails and<br>hair. | Do not use on<br>face or skin<br>creases. May<br>stain fabric, skin,<br>or hair. | Apply with<br>plastic gloves.<br>Remove by<br>washing. | Used to treat<br>psoriasis. |
| **Chlorhexidine**<br>*Hibiclens* scrub,<br>cleanser (OTC) | Irritation, rash,<br>burning. | | | Used as an<br>antiseptic and<br>germicide. |
| **Hexachlorophene**<br>*pHisoHex* scrub,<br>cleanser (℞) | Irritation, rash,<br>burning. | | | Used as an<br>antiseptic and<br>germicide. |
| **Hydroquinone**<br>*Eldopaque, Solaquin*<br>cream (OTC)<br>*Melanex* solution<br>(℞) | Dryness,<br>erythema, sting-<br>ing, dermatitis. | Protect skin<br>from the sun. | | Used for bleach-<br>ing of hyperpig-<br>mented skin. |

Miscellaneous

**ACTION** These products work by a variety of mechanism to affect skin coloring, tone, elasticity, pain, dryness, and removal of dead skin.

**INDICATION** These products are used for dandruff, psoriasis, seborrhea, and burns, and as anesthetics, analgesics, antihistamines, antiseptics, and liniments.

| Generic Name<br>*Brand Name* | Side Effects | Warnings | Dosing | Notes |
|---|---|---|---|---|
| **Imiquimod**<br>*Aldara* cream (℞) | Edema, erythema, erosion. | Do not cover after applying medication. | Apply at bedtime and wash off in the morning. | Used for treatment of genital and perianal warts. |
| **Mafenide**<br>*Sulfamylon* cream (℞) | Rash, itching, edema. | Notify physician if hyperventilation occurs. | | Used for treatment of second and third degree burns. |
| **Methoxsalen**<br>*Oxsoralen* lotion (℞) | Skin burns. | Avoid sun exposure. | | Used to treat severe psoriasis in conjunction with UV radiation. |
| **Nitrofurazone**<br>*Furacin* ointment, cream (℞) | Rash, pruritus, local edema. | Avoid exposure to direct sunlight and excessive heat. | | For second and third degree burns and bacterial infections. |
| **Minoxidil**<br>*Rogaine* solution (OTC) | Irritation, rash, burning, chest pain, blood pressure changes, nausea, vomiting. | For external use only. Ingestion of solution could produce severe adverse effects. | Apply only to healthy scalp. | Used to treat male pattern baldness and for diffuse hair loss in females. |
| **Podofilox**<br>*Condylox* solution (℞) | Burning, pain, inflammation, erosion, itching. | Allow to dry well after application before allowing other skin surfaces to touch. | Apply with cotton-tipped applicator. | Used for treatment of genital warts. |
| **Povidone-Iodine**<br>*Betadine* ointment, solution, other dosage forms (OTC) | Irritation, rash, burning. | | | Used as an antiseptic and germicide. |
| **Selenium Sulfide**<br>*Selsun Blue* shampoo (OTC)<br>*Selsun, Exsel* shampoo (℞) | Skin irritation, hair discoloration, hair loss. | Avoid contact with eyes. Do not use on inflamed skin. | | Used to treat dandruff, seborrheic dermatitis, and tinea versicolor. |

**ACTION** These products work by a variety of mechanism to affect skin coloring, tone, elasticity, pain, dryness, and removal of dead skin.

**INDICATION** These products are used for dandruff, psoriasis, seborrhea, and burns, and as anesthetics, analgesics, antihistamines, antiseptics, and liniments.

| Generic Name<br>*Brand Name* | Side Effects | Warnings | Dosing | Notes |
|---|---|---|---|---|
| **Silver Sulfadiazine**<br>*Silvadene, SSD*<br>cream (℞) | Burning, itching, kidney inflammation. | | Apply with sterile gloves. | Used to prevent and treat bacterial infection in second and third degree burns. |

# Vaginal Products

**ACTION** These medications kill bacteria by preventing the formation of the normal cell bacterial wall, thereby increasing the likelihood that the cell will rupture.

**INDICATION** Used to treat vaginal infections caused by fungi or bacteria. It is important to take the full course of therapy to prevent a recurrence of the infection.

| Generic Name<br>*Brand Name* | Side Effects | Warnings | Dosing | Notes |
|---|---|---|---|---|
| **Butoconazole Nitrate**<br>*Femstat* vaginal cream (OTC) | Vaginal swelling, discharge, soreness. | May weaken latex or rubber products such as condoms or diaphragms. | Do not engage in vaginal sexual intercourse during treatment or male partner should use a condom to avoid risk of reinfection. Complete full course of therapy. | Used for the treatment of vaginal candidiasis (yeast) infection. |
| **Clindamycin Phosphate**<br>*Cleocin* vaginal cream (℞) | Burning, itching, irritation. Contact a doctor if these persist. | May weaken latex or rubber products such as condoms or diaphragms. | Do not engage in vaginal sexual intercourse during treatment. Complete full course of therapy. | Used for the treatment of bacterial infections. |

**ACTION** These medications kill bacteria by preventing the formation of the normal cell bacterial wall, thereby increasing the likelihood that the cell will rupture.

**INDICATION** Used to treat vaginal infections caused by fungi or bacteria. It is important to take the full course of therapy to prevent a recurrence of the infection.

| Generic Name *Brand Name* | Side Effects | Warnings | Dosing | Notes |
|---|---|---|---|---|
| **Clotrimazole** *Femcare, Gyne-Lotrimin, Mycelex-7* vaginal cream, tablets (OTC) *Mycelex-G* vaginal tablets (℞) | Abdominal cramps, bloating, vaginal rash, painful intercourse. | May weaken latex or rubber products such as condoms or diaphragms. | Do not engage in vaginal sexual intercourse during treatment. Complete full course of therapy. | Used for the treatment of Candida albicans yeast infections only. |
| **Metronidazole** *MetroGel* vaginal gel (℞) | Burning, itching, irritation. Contact a doctor if these persist. | May weaken latex or rubber products such as condoms or diaphragms. | Do not engage in vaginal sexual intercourse during treatment. Complete full course of therapy. | Used for the treatment of bacterial vaginosis. |
| **Miconazole Nitrate** *Monistat* vaginal cream, suppository (OTC, ℞) | Pelvic cramps, headache, hives, skin rash. | May weaken latex or rubber products such as condoms or diaphragms. | Do not engage in vaginal sexual intercourse during treatment. Complete full course of therapy. | Used for the treatment of Candida albicans yeast infections only. |
| **Nystatin** *Mycostatin* vaginal tablet (℞) | Irritation, rash. | May weaken latex or rubber products such as condoms or diaphragms. | Do not engage in vaginal sexual intercourse during treatment. Complete full course of therapy. | Used for the treatment of Candida albicans yeast infections only. |
| **Oxytetracycline, Polymyxin B Sulfate** *Terramycin with Polymyxin* vaginal tablet (℞) | Burning, itching, irritation. Contact a doctor if these persist. | May weaken latex or rubber products such as condoms or diaphragms. | Do not engage in vaginal sexual intercourse during treatment. Complete full course of therapy. | Used for the treatment of bacterial vaginal infections. |

**ACTION** These medications kill bacteria by preventing the formation of the normal cell bacterial wall, thereby increasing the likelihood that the cell will rupture.

**INDICATION** Used to treat vaginal infections caused by fungi or bacteria. It is important to take the full course of therapy to prevent a recurrence of the infection.

| Generic Name *Brand Name* | Side Effects | Warnings | Dosing | Notes |
|---|---|---|---|---|
| **Sulfanilamide** *AVC* vaginal cream, suppository (℞) | Burning, itching, irritation. Contact a doctor if these persist. | May weaken latex or rubber products such as condoms or diaphragms. | Do not engage in vaginal sexual intercourse during treatment. Complete full course of therapy. | Used for the treatment of Candida albicans yeast infections only. |
| **Terconazole** *Terazol* vaginal cream, suppository (℞) | Headache, body aches, sensitivity to light, painful menstruation, abdominal pain, fever. | May weaken latex or rubber products such as condoms or diaphragms. | Do not engage in vaginal sexual intercourse during treatment. Complete full course of therapy. | Used for the treatment of Candida albicans yeast infections only. |
| **Tioconazole** *Vagistat-1* vaginal ointment (OTC) | Vaginal discharge, pain, dryness, scaling, excessive urination at night, painful intercourse. | May weaken latex or rubber products such as condoms or diaphragms. | Do not engage in vaginal sexual intercourse during treatment. Complete full course of therapy. | Used for the treatment of Candida albicans yeast infections only. |
| **Triple Sulfa** *Sultrin* vaginal tablet (℞) *Gyne-Sulf, Sultrin, Trysul* vaginal cream (℞) | Burning, itching, irritation. Contact a doctor if these persist. | May weaken latex or rubber products such as condoms or diaphragms. | Do not engage in vaginal sexual intercourse during treatment. Complete full course of therapy. | Used for the treatment of bacterial vaginosis. |

# Schedule of Controlled Substances

The Drug Enforcement Agency (DEA) regulates the manufacturing, distribution, and prescribing of drugs that have a potential for abuse. The schedule of controlled substances categorizes dugs according to the degree of medical use and abuse potential. This list is provided as a guide. State laws may have stricter regulations.

### Schedule I

High abuse potential and no accepted medical use. Includes drugs such as ecstasy, heroin, LSD, marijuana, mescaline, methaqualone, PCP (phencyclidine), peyote, and psilocybin.

### Schedule II

High abuse potential with severe dependence liability. Includes narcotics, amphetamines, and barbiturates.

### Schedule III

Lower abuse potential than Schedule II drugs and moderate dependence liability. Includes nonbarbiturate sedatives, nonamphetamine stimulants, androgenic steroids, and limited amounts of certain narcotics.

### Schedule IV

Lower abuse potential than Schedule III and limited dependence liability. Includes some sedatives, antianxiety agents, and nonnarcotic analgesics.

### Schedule V

Limited abuse potential and includes primarily small amounts of narcotics used as an antitussive or antidiarrheal.

# Record-Keeping Forms

| | Initials | | | | | | | | | | | | | | | | | | |
|---|---|---|---|---|---|---|---|---|---|---|---|---|---|---|---|---|---|---|---|
| | **# of Packets** | | | | | | | | | | | | | | | | | | |
| I-Prin | | | | | | | | | | | | | | | | | | | |
| Aleve | | | | | | | | | | | | | | | | | | | |
| Aldroxicon Liquid | | | | | | | | | | | | | | | | | | | |
| Sudadrin-Forte | | | | | | | | | | | | | | | | | | | |
| CCP-Caffeine-Free | | | | | | | | | | | | | | | | | | | |
| Alamag-Plus | | | | | | | | | | | | | | | | | | | |
| APAP-Plus | | | | | | | | | | | | | | | | | | | |
| Tri-Buffered Aspirin | | | | | | | | | | | | | | | | | | | |
| Sepasoothe | | | | | | | | | | | | | | | | | | | |
| Gualcon-DMS | | | | | | | | | | | | | | | | | | | |
| Medikoff Drops | | | | | | | | | | | | | | | | | | | |
| Diphen | | | | | | | | | | | | | | | | | | | |
| Nausatrol | | | | | | | | | | | | | | | | | | | |
| Chlorphen | | | | | | | | | | | | | | | | | | | |
| Medicidin-D | | | | | | | | | | | | | | | | | | | |
| Medi-Synol | | | | | | | | | | | | | | | | | | | |
| Dio-Tame Tablets | | | | | | | | | | | | | | | | | | | |
| Diotame Liquid | | | | | | | | | | | | | | | | | | | |
| Diamode | | | | | | | | | | | | | | | | | | | |
| Medi-lyte | | | | | | | | | | | | | | | | | | | |
| | **Name** | | | | | | | | | | | | | | | | | | |
| | **Date** | | | | | | | | | | | | | | | | | | |

| Date | Name | Drug Dispensed | Number/<br>Packets | Initials |
|------|------|----------------|--------------------|----------|
|      |      |                |                    |          |
|      |      |                |                    |          |
|      |      |                |                    |          |
|      |      |                |                    |          |
|      |      |                |                    |          |
|      |      |                |                    |          |
|      |      |                |                    |          |
|      |      |                |                    |          |
|      |      |                |                    |          |
|      |      |                |                    |          |
|      |      |                |                    |          |
|      |      |                |                    |          |
|      |      |                |                    |          |
|      |      |                |                    |          |
|      |      |                |                    |          |
|      |      |                |                    |          |
|      |      |                |                    |          |
|      |      |                |                    |          |
|      |      |                |                    |          |
|      |      |                |                    |          |
|      |      |                |                    |          |
|      |      |                |                    |          |
|      |      |                |                    |          |
|      |      |                |                    |          |

# Poison Control Centers

**Alabama**
Alabama Poison Center
408 A. Paul Bryant Drive East
Tuscaloosa, Alabama 35401
800-462-0800

**Alaska**
Anchorage Poison Control Center
Providence Hospital Pharmacy
3200 Providence Drive, Box 796604
Anchorage, Alaska 99519-6604
800-478-3193

**Arizona**
Arizona Poison/Drug Information
  Center
University of Arizona
Arizona Health Science Center
Room 1156
1501 North Campbell Avenue
Tucson, Arizona 85724
800-362-0101

**Arkansas**
Arkansas Poison/Drug Information
Center College of Pharmacy
4301 West Markham Street
Little Rock, Arkansas 72205
800-376-4766

**California**
Los Angeles Regional Drug
  and Poison Information Center
LAC–USC Medical Center
1200 N. State Street—
  Rm GH 1107
Los Angeles, California 90033
800-825-2722

**Colorado**
Rocky Mountain Poison/Drug Center
645 Bannock Street
Denver, Colorado 80204-4507
800-332-3073

**Connecticut**
Connecticut Poison Control Center
University of Connecticut Health
  Center
263 Farmington Avenue
Farmington, Connecticut 06030
800-343-2722

**Delaware**
The Poison Control Center
3600 Science Center, Suite 220
Philadelphia, Pennsylvania 19104-
  2643
800-722-7112

**District of Columbia**
National Capital Poison Center
3201 New Mexico Avenue, NW
Suite 310
Washington, DC 20016
800-498-8666

**Florida**
Florida Poison Information Center
PO Box 1289
Tampa General Hospital
Tampa, Florida 33601
800-282-3171

**Georgia**
Georgia Poison Center
Hughes Spalding Children's Hospital
Grady Health Systems
80 Butler Street, SE
PO Box 26066
Atlanta, Georgia 30335-3801
800-282-5846

**Hawaii**
Hawaii Poison Center
Kapiolani Women's and Children
    Medical Center
1319 Punahou Street
Honolulu, Hawaii 96826
800-362-3585

**Idaho**
Idaho Poison Center
3092 Elder Street
Boise, Idaho 83705
800-632-8000

**Illinois**
Swedish-American Regional Poison
Resource Center
Swedish-American Hospital
1400 Charles Street
Rockford, Illinois 61104
800-252-2022

**Indiana**
Indiana Poison Center
Methodist Hospital of Indiana
I-65 & 21st Street
PO Box 1367
Indianapolis, Indiana 46206-1367
800-382-9097

**Iowa**
Poison Control Center
University of Iowa Hospital/Clinics
200 Hawkins Drive
Iowa City, Iowa 52242
800-272-6477

**Kansas**
Mid-American Poison Control
    Center
University of Kansas Medical
    Center
3901 Rainbow Boulevard,
    Room B-400
Kansas City, Kansas 66160-7231
800-332-6633

**Kentucky**
Kentucky Regional Poison Center
Kosair Children's Hospital
234 East Gray Street
PO Box 35070
Louisville, Kentucky 40232-5070
800-722-5725

**Louisiana**
Louisiana Drug and Poison Center
Northeast Louisiana University
    School of Pharmacy, Sugar Hall
Monroe, Louisiana 71209-6430
800-256-9822

**Maine**
Maine Poison Control Center
Maine Medical Center
22 Bramhall Street
Portland, Maine 04102
800-442-6305

**Maryland**
Maryland Poison Center
University of Maryland School of
    Pharmacy
20 North Pine Street
Baltimore, Maryland 21201
800-492-2414

**Massachusetts**
Massachusetts Poison Control
    System
The Children's Hospital
300 Longwood Avenue
Boston, Massachusetts 02115
800-682-9211

**Michigan**
Poison Control Center
Children's Hospital of Michigan
3901 Beaubian Boulevard
Detroit, Michigan 48201
800-745-5711

**Minnesota**
Minnesota Regional Poison Center
St. Paul-Ramsey Medical Center
640 Jackson Street
St. Paul, Minnesota 55101
800-222-1222

**Mississippi**
Mississippi Regional Poison Center
University of Mississippi Medical
    Center
2500 North State Street
Jackson, Mississippi 39216
601-354-7660

**Missouri**
Cardinal Glennon
    Children's Hospital
Regional Poison Center
1465 South Grand Boulevard
St. Louis, Missouri 63104
800-366-8888

**Montana**
Rocky Mountain Poison/Drug
    Center
645 Bannock Street
Denver, CO 80204-4507
800-332-3073

**Nebraska**
The Poison Center
Children's Memorial Hospital
8301 Dodge Street
Omaha, Nebraska 68114
800-955-9119

**Nevada**
Humana Hospital Sunrise
3186 Maryland Parkway
Las Vegas, Nevada 89109
800-446-6179

**New Hampshire**
New Hampshire Poison
    Information Center
Dartmouth-Hitchcock Memorial
    Hospital
1 Medical Center Drive
Lebanon, New Hampshire 03756
800-764-7661

**New Jersey**
New Jersey Poison Information
201 Lyons Avenue
Newark, New Jersey 07112
800-962-1253

**New Mexico**
New Mexico Poison/Drug Center
University of New Mexico
2400 Marble Street
Albuquerque, New Mexico
    87131-1076
800-432-6866

**New York**
Central New York Poison Control
    Center
SUNY Health Science Center
750 East Adams Street
Syracuse, New York 13210

**North Carolina**
Carolinas Poison Center
Carolinas Medical Center
1000 Blythe Boulevard
Charlotte, North Carolina
    28232-2861

**North Dakota**
North Dakota Poison Information
    Center
720 4th Street North
Fargo, North Dakota 58122
800-732-2200

**Ohio**
Central Ohio Poison Control Center
700 Childrens Drive
Columbus, Ohio 43205-2696
800-682-7625

**Oklahoma**
Oklahoma Poison Control Center
Children's Memorial Hospital
940 NE 13th Street
Oklahoma City, Oklahoma 73104
800-522-4611

**Oregon**
Oregon Poison Center
Oregon Health Sciences University
3181 SW Sam Jackson Park Road
Portland, Oregon 97201
800-452-7165

**Pennsylvania**
Central Pennsylvania Poison Center
Milton S. Hershey Medical Center
University Drive, PO Box 850
Hershey, Pennsylvania 17033
800-521-6110

**Puerto Rico**
Drug Information Center
University of Puerto Rico
College of Pharmacy
GPO Box 5067
San Juan, Puerto Rico 00936
809-736-0196

**Rhode Island**
Rhode Island Poison Center
593 Eddy Street
Providence, Rhode Island
401-444-5727

**South Carolina**
Palmetto Poison Center
University of South Carolina
College of Pharmacy
Columbia, South Carolina 29208
800-922-1117

**South Dakota**
McKennan Poison Center
McKennan Hospital
800 E. 21st Street
Sioux Falls, South Dakota
57117-5045
800-952-0123

**Tennessee**
Middle Tennessee Regional Poison
  Center
1161 21st Avenue South
501 Oxford House
Nashville, Tennessee 37232-4632
800-288-9999

**Texas**
North Texas Poison Center
Parkland Memorial Hospital
5201 Harry Hines Boulevard
PO Box 35926
Dallas, Texas 75235
800-441-0040

**Utah**
Utah Poison Control Center
410 Chipeta Way, Suite 230
Salt Lake City, Utah 84108
800-456-7707

**Vermont**
Vermont Poison Center
111 Colchester Avenue
Burlington, Vermont 05401
802-658-3456

**Virginia**
Blue Ridge Poison Center
University of Virginia Health
  Sciences Center Box 67
Charlottesville, Virginia 22901
800-451-1428

**Washington**
Washington Poison Center
155 NE 100th Street, Suite 400
Seattle, Washington 98125-8012
800-732-6985

**West Virginia**
West Virginia Poison Center
3110 MacCorkle Avenue SE
Charleston, West Virginia 25304
800-642-3625

**Wisconsin**
Regional Poison Center
University of Wisconsin Hospital
F6/133 CSC
600 Highland Avenue
Madison, Wisconsin 53792
608-262-3702

**Wyoming**
The Poison Center
c/o Mid-Plains Poison Center
8301 Dodge Street
Omaha, Nebraska 68114
402-390-5555

# Common Terms and Definitions

**Administer:** to provide one dose of a drug; the drug is taken at time of administration

**Agonist:** substance that stimulates or facilitates a reaction at a specific site

**Allergy:** state of hypersensitivity to a foreign substance manifested by an exaggerated response of the immune system

**Analgesic:** substance that decreases or relieves pain

**Anaphylactic shock:** state of shock caused by an allergic reaction

**Anesthesia:** partial or total loss of sensation

**Antacid:** substance used to neutralize excess acid in the stomach

**Antagonist:** substance that inhibits or blocks a reaction at a specific site

**Antianxiety:** prevents or relieves anxiety/nervousness

**Antibiotic:** substance that prevents, inhibits, or destroys life

**Anticoagulant:** substance that decreases the capacity of the blood to coagulate

**Antidepressant:** substance that relieves or prevents psychic depression

**Antidiarrheal:** relieves or prevents diarrhea

**Antidiuretic:** substance that decreases the formation of urine

**Antidote:** substance that relieves, prevents, or counteracts the effects of poison

**Antiemetic:** substance that inhibits vomiting

**Antifungal:** treats infections caused by fungal agents

**Antihistamine:** compound that counteracts histamine in the body; used to treat allergic reactions and cold symptoms

**Antihypertensive:** acts against high blood pressure

**Anti-inflammatory:** decreases inflammation

**Antipsychotic:** alleviates psychosis or psychotic states

**Antipyretic:** reduces fever

**Antiseptic:** stops the growth of germs; used on surface of skin to prevent infections of superficial wounds

**Antitoxic:** counteracts toxins

**Antitussive:** suppresses a cough

**Anxiolytic:** relieves anxiety

**Asthma:** chronic disease of the respiratory system characterized by bronchoconstriction, airway inflammation, and formation of mucous plugs in the airway

**Antispasmodic:** prevents or relieves spasms

**Bronchitis:** inflammatory condition of the mucosal lining of the tracheobronchial tree characterized by bronchial swelling, mucus secretions, and cilia dysfunction

**Bronchospasm:** contraction of the smooth muscles of the bronchial tubes causing narrowing of the airway

**Bronchodilator:** substance that opens the bronchial tubes of the lungs to increase the flow of air

**Caustic:** chemical action that destroys or eats away at a substance

**Conjunctivitis:** bacterial infection characterized by itching, burning, watering, and eye inflammation; pinkeye

**Constipation:** condition characterized by infrequent or incomplete bowel movements

**Corticosteroids:** group of cortisone-like hormones that are secreted by the adrenal cortex and are critical to body functions

**Counterirritant:** substance that produces superficial irritation with the object of reducing another irritation

**Cystitis:** urethra or bladder inflammation, characterized by discomfort during urination

**Decongestant:** substance that relieves congestion

**Depressant:** substance that reduces bodily function or an instinctive desire

**Diabetes:** metabolic disorder characterized by near or absolute lack of insulin, insulin resistance, or both

**Diarrhea:** condition characterized by loose or watery stool

**Dispense:** to provide a dose or more than a dose of a drug to be taken later than at the time of dispensing

**Depressant:** substance that decreases the functioning of the central nervous system and other bodily functions

**Diuretic:** substance that increases the flow of urine

**Dosage:** amount of medication that is used for treating a given condition or illness

**Dose:** amount of medication that is administered at one time to produce a specific effect

**Drug:** any substance that produces a functional change in the body

**Drug administration:** providing one dose of a specific drug

**Drug dispensing:** providing more than one dose of a specific drug

**Dysmennorhea:** condition characterized by difficult or painful menstruation; menstrual cramps

**Dysuria:** condition characterized by pain or burning sensation and difficulty during urination

**Emetic:** substance that initiates or facilitates vomiting

**Enteric coated:** coating on tablets that allows them to pass through stomach unchanged before being broken down in small intestine and absorbed; used to protect stomach from medicines or the medicine from stomach acids

**Expectorant:** substance that promotes the discharge or expulsion of mucus from the respiratory tract

**Gastroenteritis:** condition characterized by inflammation of the mucous membrane of the stomach and/or small intestine

**Generic:** general name of drug substance, not owned by specific group as a trademark or brand name

**Germicide:** substance that destroys germs

**Hemorrhoids:** condition characterized by rectal and anal dilations of the venous plexus that can become exposed if they protrude internally or externally

**Histamine:** chemical produced by cells; involved in the mediation of certain physiological responses as well as hypersensitivity responses; allergic responses

**Hyperglycemia:** condition characterized by abnormally high levels of glucose in the circulating blood that can lead to diabetic coma

**Hypertension:** condition characterized by sustained elevated blood pressure

**Hypotension:** condition characterized by sustained depression in blood pressure

**Hypoglycemia:** condition characterized by abnormally low levels of glucose in the circulating blood that can lead to insulin shock

**Idiosyncratic:** unexpected drug response

**Infection:** invasion of a host or host tissue by a foreign substance such as bacteria, fungi, or viruses and characterized by swelling, redness, and localized elevated temperature

**Inflammation:** pain, swelling, redness, heat, and loss of function that accompany musculoskeletal injuries

**Influenza:** acute infectious respiratory tract condition characterized by malaise, headache, dry cough, and general muscle aches

**Inhalant:** substance that enters the body through inhaling

**Irritant:** something that irritates or excites

**Laxatives:** substance that promotes peristalsis and evacuation of the bowel in a relatively slow manner

**Meningitis:** condition characterized by inflammation of the meninges of the brain and spinal column

**Migraine:** condition characterized by throbbing headache, usually affecting one side of the head; often accompanied by nausea, vomiting, and sensitivity to light

**Myositis:** inflammation of connective tissue within a muscle

**Narcotic:** substance that dulls the senses, relieves pain, and induces profound sleep, but in excessive doses causes stupor, coma, or convulsions

**Oral:** relating to the mouth

**Otitis externa:** bacterial infection involving the lining of the auditory canal; swimmer's ear

**Otitis media:** localized infection in the middle ear secondary to upper respiratory infections

**Pharmacodynamics:** study of how drugs affect the body

**Pharmacokinetics:** study of how the body absorbs, distributes, metabolizes, and excretes drugs

**Pharmacology:** study of drugs

**Pharmacotherapeutics:** study of how drugs are used in the prevention and treatment of disease

**Pharmacy:** professional discipline of the preparation and dispensing of medications

**Pharmacology:** study of drugs

**Pharyngitis:** viral, bacterial, or fungal infection of the pharynx leading to a sore throat

**Potency:** dosage of a drug that produces a given responses in a specific amplitude

**Prognosis:** probable course or progression of an injury or disease

**Rhinitis:** condition characterized by inflammation of the nasal membranes with excessive mucus production resulting in nasal congestion

**Sedative:** substance that calms, moderates, or tranquilizes nervousness or excitement

**Serous otitis:** condition characterized by fluid buildup behind the eardrum associated with otitis media and upper respiratory infections

**Side effect:** effect produced by a drug that occurs in addition to the main therapeutic response

**Sinusitis:** condition characterized by inflammation of the paranasal sinuses

**Stimulant:** substance that increases the functioning of the central nervous system and other bodily functions

**Sublingual:** under the tongue

**Suppository:** mass of medicated material shaped for insertion into the rectum, vagina, or urethra

**Tinea:** ringworm; fungal infection of the hair, skin, or nails characterized by small vesicles, itching, and scaling

**Tinea capitis:** ringworm of the scalp

**Tinea cruris:** fungal infection of groin area; jock itch

**Tinea pedis:** fungal infection of feet and toes; athlete's foot

**Tolerance:** acquired phenomenon associated with some drugs in which larger doses of the drug are needed to achieve a given response when the drug is used for prolonged periods

**Topical:** produces local effects when applied directly to the skin

**Toxic:** poisonous; related to or caused by a toxin

**Toxicology:** study of the harmful effects of drugs

**Vaccination:** substance, typically consisting of modified infectious microorganisms, which is administered to prevent disease

**Vasoconstrictor:** substance that constricts blood vessels, decreasing blood flow

**Vasodilator:** substance that dilates blood vessels, permitting increased blood flow

**Vertigo:** balance disturbance characterized by a whirling sensation of oneself or external objects

## REFERENCES

Anderson MK, Hall SJ. Sports Injury Management. Baltimore, MD: Williams & Wilkins, 1995.

Ciccone CD. Pharmacology in Rehabilitation. Philadelphia: F. A. Davis, 1990.

Drug Facts and Comparisons. St. Louis, MO: Facts and Comparison, 1996.

Gean CJ, Meyers FH. Pocket Drug Guide. 2nd ed. Baltimore, MD: Williams & Wilkins, 1996.

Handbook of Prescription Drugs. 9th ed. Washington, DC: American Pharmaceutical Association, 1995.

Herbert DL. Dispensing prescription medications to athletes. In: Herbert DL, ed. The Legal Aspects of Sports Medicine. Canton, OH: Professional Sports Publications, 1991: 215–224.

NCAA Guideline 1c: Dispensing Prescription Medication. June 1992.

Patient Drug Facts. St. Louis, MO: Facts and Comparisons, 1996.

Prentice WE, Huff PS. Pharmacological considerations in a rehabilitation program. In: Prentice WE, ed. Rehabilitation Techniques in Sports Medicine. 2nd ed. St. Louis: Mosby, 1994: 220–237.

Price KD, Huff PS, Isetts BJ, Goldwire MA. University-based sports pharmacy program. American Journal of Health-System Pharmacists. 1995; 52:302–309.

Stedman's Concise Medical Dictionary. 2nd ed. Baltimore, MD: Williams & Wilkins, 1993.

USP-DI. United States Pharmacoepia, 1996.

Webster's Ninth New Collegiate Dictionary. Springfield, MA: Merriam-Webster, 1991.